Lynda Aoudia

Malignant breast tumors

Lynda Aoudia

Malignant breast tumors

Correlations between imaging and histological types

ScienciaScripts

Imprint

Cover image: www.ingimage.com

This book is a translation from the original published under ISBN 978-620-6-71298-5.

Publisher:
Sciencia Scripts
is a trademark of
Dodo Books Indian Ocean Ltd. and OmniScriptum S.R.L publishing group

120 High Road, East Finchley, London, N2 9ED, United Kingdom
Str. Armeneasca 28/1, office 1, Chisinau MD-2012, Republic of Moldova, Europe
Printed at: see last page
ISBN: 978-620-7-68156-3

Malignant breast tumors

Correlations between imaging and histological types

Lynda AOUDIA

Foreword

Breast cancer is the most common cancer in women worldwide. The histological type of tumor according to the WHO is an essential morphological diagnostic and prognostic element in the management of breast cancer.

The aim of this book is to explain the various mammographic, ultrasound and MRI aspects of the different histological types of breast cancer, and to highlight some of the particular imaging features of these histological types.

Prof. Lynda AOUDIA

Table of contents

Introduction

Breast cancer is the leading cancer in women worldwide. In 15 years, incidence has increased by 50% [1]. Over the same period, the number of deaths has risen by only 17%, reflecting progress in breast cancer screening and therapeutic advances.

Imaging is used at every stage in the management of this pathology, in screening, diagnosis, extension assessment, follow-up under treatment and post-treatment monitoring. It can also help predict the histological types of breast cancer, in order to guide management.

Numerous studies address the imaging aspects of each tumor type that radiologists need to be aware of.

Anatomical reminder

1. Breast anatomy

The breast is a globular organ occupying the anterosuperior part of the thorax. It is located above the pectoralis muscle, which provides support [2]. It consists mainly of a mammary gland, supportive connective tissue and adipose tissue, all covered by the skin. The apex of the breast is represented by the nipple surrounded by the areola (fig. 1). It is made up of some fifteen main galactophores, each delimiting a lobe. The milk ducts open into the nipple at the level of the milk pores, after dilating slightly to form a lactiferous sinus.

Thin fibrous partitions separate the lobes, extending from the anterior surface of the gland into the dermis to form Cooper's ligaments and Duret's ridges (fig. 1).

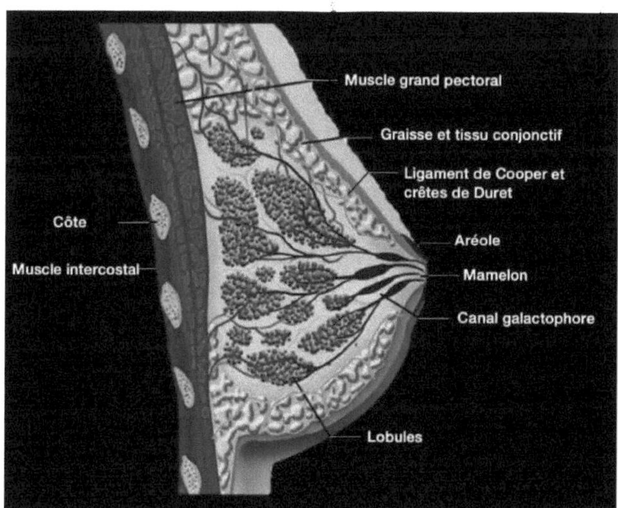

Fig. 1. anatomical structure of the breast.

2. Galactophoric tree

The breast is made up of some fifteen main milk ducts, which end in a nipple pore. These main ducts, after a dilatation known as the lactiferous sinus, branch out into secondary ducts of medium and small caliber up to the Ductulo-Lobular Terminal Unit (DLTU).

This UDTL consists of an extra- and intra-lobular terminal galactophore and a lobule made up of ten or so alveoli called acini. The UDTL is embedded in a loose connective tissue known as pallaeal tissue. All this tissue is surrounded by adipose tissue (fig. 2).

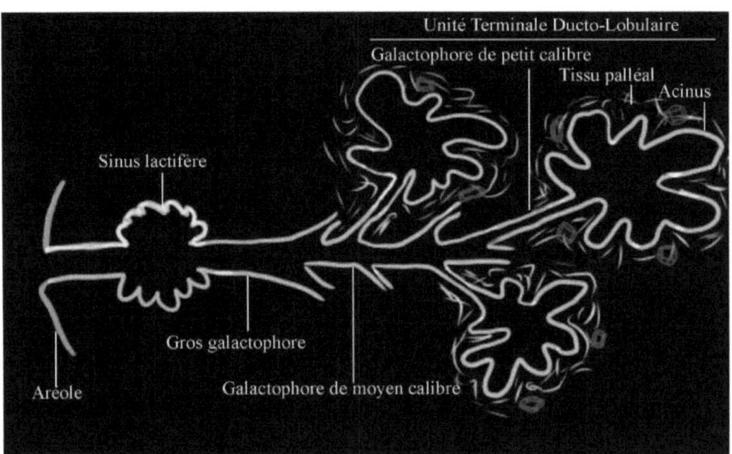

Fig. 2: Diagram of the galactophoric tree.

Histological reminder

The entire galactophoric tree is made up of a double cell bed resting on a basement membrane in direct contact with the blood vessels (fig. 3):

- an inner layer of columnar epithelial cells, responsible for the milk secretory function.
- an outer layer of myoepithelial cells responsible for contraction.

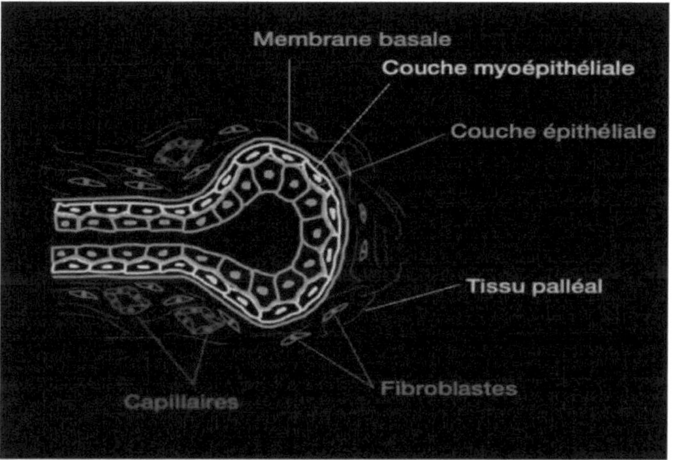

Fig. 3: Histological diagram of acinar constituents.

Histopathological background

Around 95% of malignant tumours are carcinomas, meaning that they develop from the epithelial cells of the mammary ducts and lobules. Sarcomas and lymphomas are rare, and intramammary metastases exceptional [3].

Breast cancer stage

There are several stages in the development of breast cancer: carcinoma in situ and infiltrating carcinoma (fig. 4).

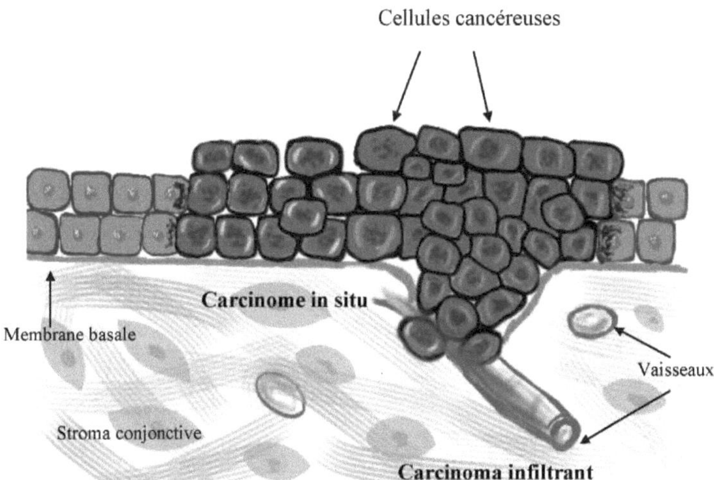

Fig. 4. in situ and invasive breast carcinoma.

1. Carcinoma in situ

In situ cancer is defined as the proliferation of malignant tumour cells confined to the interior of normal epithelial structures, which have not crossed the basement membrane, without metastatic potential.

2. Invasive carcinoma

Infiltrating carcinoma is a cell proliferation which, having crossed the basement membrane, infiltrates the surrounding breast tissue. There are more than twenty-two (22) histological entities recognized by the WHO, and two main groups can be distinguished: the non-specific form, formerly known as infiltrating ductal carcinoma, which accounts for around two-thirds of all infiltrating cancers, and the other so-called specific forms [3] (table 1) (appendix 1).

Table 1. WHO classification		
WHO classification 2012		**WHO classification 2003**
Nonspecific carcinoma (NST) 80% of cases Type-specific carcinoma:		**-Invasive ductal carcinoma** Lobular carcinoma
Lobular carcinoma	5-15%	Tubular carcinoma Cribriform carcinoma Mucinous carcinoma Micropapillary carcinoma Metaplastic carcinoma
Tubular carcinoma Cribriform carcinoma mucinous carcinoma Micropapillary carcinoma Metaplastic carcinoma **Rare types :** Secretory carcinoma Salivary gland tumors	5%	

Imaging techniques

1. Mammography

Mammography is the reference radiological examination for screening for breast cancer, the leading cause of death in women.

Mammographic images must be optimized in terms of spatial resolution, contrast and noise. A number of technical criteria need to be taken into account, including high contrast for good visualization of microcalcifications. The radiation spectrum must be broad, to adapt to varying breast densities, and the radiation dose must be minimal, especially in young patients.

1.1. Impact

Positioning the breast is a fundamental step in mammography, and the technique must be beyond reproach. The aim is to radiograph the entire mammary gland, including the deep planes. Positioning is the key to obtaining optimal images, essential for interpretation, and meeting a number of quality criteria [4].

1.1.1. Fundamental impacts

1.1.1.1.Cranio-caudal or frontal incision

The X-ray beam approaches the breast craniocaudally (fig. 5).

The difficulty of the front view lies in the absence of visualization of the deep mammary planes, and it is important to engage as much posterior mammary tissue as possible.

The criteria for successful incidence are (fig. 6):

- The breast is at the center of the image.
- The gland is well spread out.

- The nipple is at its zenith [5].
- No folds or overlaps.

The pectoralis muscle is visible in almost 30% of cases, and its presence on the x-ray allows optimum depth gain [4].

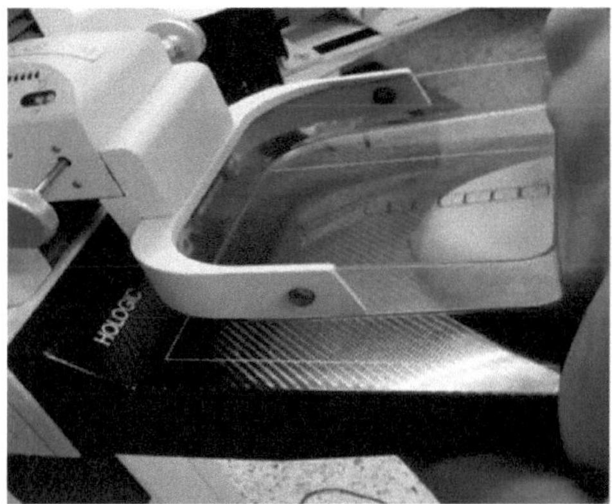

Fig. 5. Front incision.

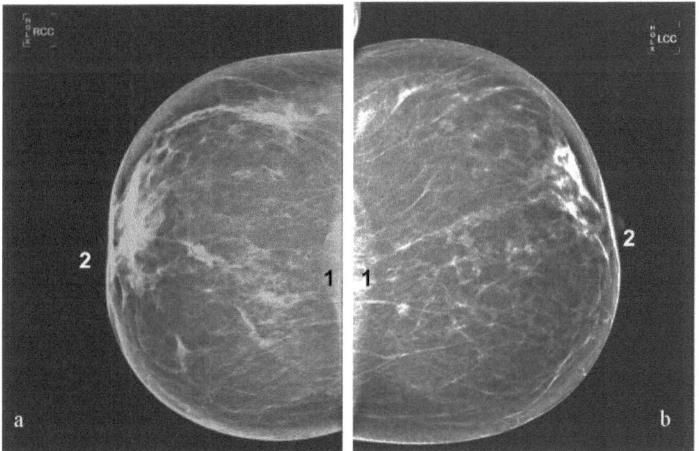

Fig. 6: Quality criteria for frontal incidence. Mammographic images. (a) Right face. (b) Left face. Pectoral muscle (1), nipple at zenith (2).

1.1.1.2.45° external oblique incidence°

This allows the breast to be studied in its long axis, and a maximum amount of breast tissue to be analyzed [6]. The stand is tilted at a strict 45°° to ensure reproducible incidence (fig. 7).

The difficulty with this incidence is to evenly compress the pectoral muscle, the breast and the submammary fold.

The criteria for successful incidence are (fig. 8)

- The pectoral muscle is visible up to halfway up the image [7].
- The nipple is at its zenith, opposite the tip of the pectoral muscle [6].
- Presence of abdominal wall skin fold [5].
- The long axis of the breast tends towards the horizontal.
- Presence of the "open" submammary fold, perfectly clear of the abdominal wall [8].
- No folds or overlaps.

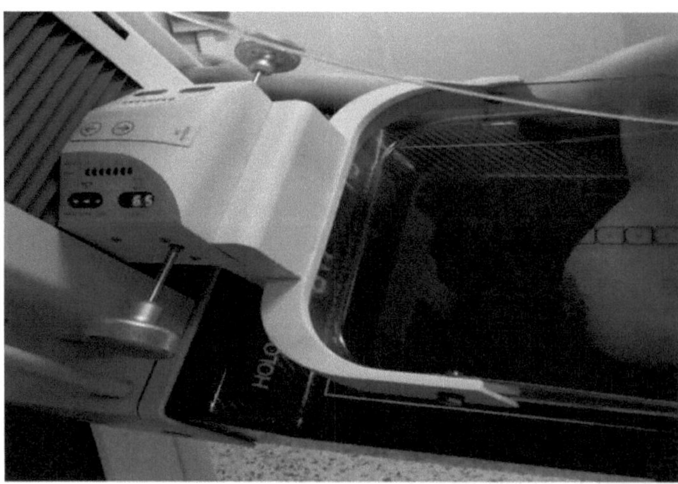

Fig. 7. External oblique incidence.

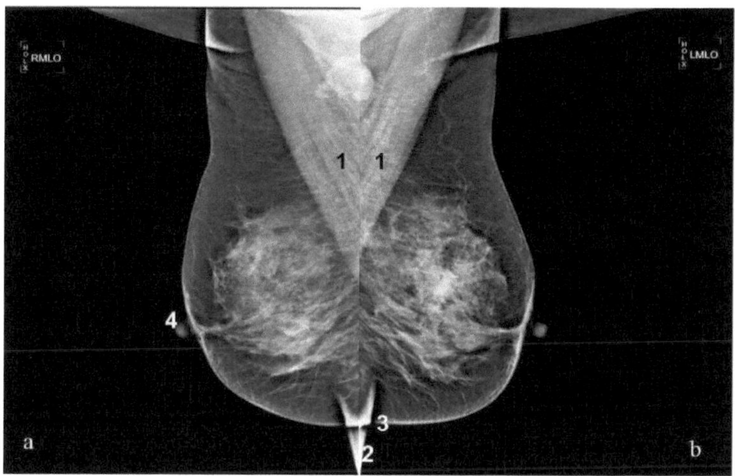

Fig. 8 Quality criteria for external oblique incidence. Mammographic images (a) Right oblique (b) Left oblique. Pectoral muscle (1), abdominal wall skin fold (2), open sub-mammary fold (3), nipple at zenith (4).

1.1.2. Additional impacts

They are always carried out in addition to the fundamental impacts.

1.1.2.1 Profile incidence

It is useful for determining the precise location of a lesion. It can also be used to highlight the sloping nature of microcalcifications.

1.1.2.2. Localized centric view

It can be used to analyze the contours of a nodule or stellar image, or to eliminate a constructed image (fig. 9).

1.1.2.3. Enlarged centered shot

Microcalcifications visible on standard images can be enlarged for detailed analysis (number, appearance, organization, etc.) (fig. 10).

1.1.2.4. Other impacts

Axillary extension, Cleopatra incidence, staggered frontal incidence, tangential cliché, Eklund maneuver [9-12].

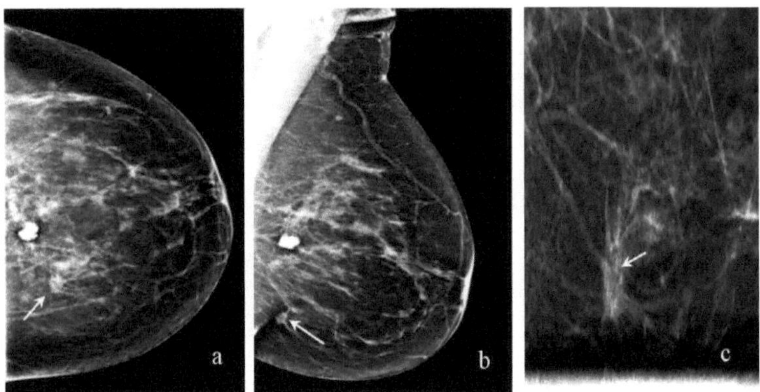

Fig. 9. localized centric view. (a) Front view. Mass with indistinct contours (arrow). (b) External oblique view. Mass in the sub mammary fold with poorly defined contours (arrow). (c). View centred on the mass. Mass with spiculated contours, BIRADS 5 (arrow).

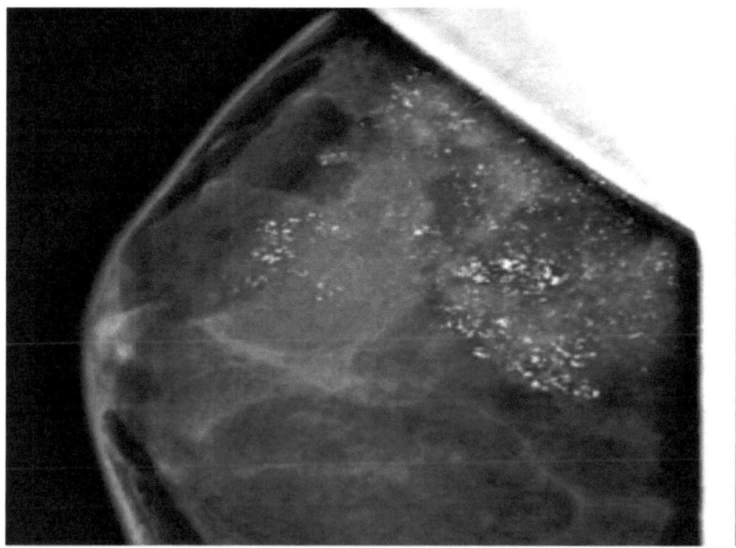

Fig. 10. Enlarged centric view. Magnification of a focus of microcalcifications.

2. Ultrasound

Ultrasound is an accessible, non-irradiating and inexpensive imaging technique. It may be indicated as a complement to mammography, to improve lesion detection, particularly in dense breasts, and to characterize lesions, notably to differentiate solid from cystic lesions, and to take samples [13].

Ultrasound of the breast is performed with a high-frequency probe, usually between 9 and 15 MHz, for good contrast and spatial resolution [14]. There are several ultrasound modes.

2.1 Mode B

This is the first technique used when performing breast ultrasound. Ultrasound waves are emitted and collected by the probe, at the same frequency, in a single direction. They are combined to create a 2D grayscale image of the breast [15]. This technique enables structures to be differentiated on the basis of the acoustic and mechanical properties of the tissue. This B-mode has a number of weaknesses, including inconsistent optimal resolution and artifacts that can degrade image quality [16] (fig. 11).

2.2. Harmonic mode

It is linked to the non-linear behavior of breast tissue with respect to ultrasound. As the ultrasound wave propagates through breast tissue, it undergoes progressive distortion of the ultrasound pulse shape, creating harmonic frequencies which are multiples of the emission frequency [17-19]. Once the initial signal has been filtered, the harmonic signal is used for image reconstruction. This technique improves the contrast of ultrasound images, particularly in the case of cysts with "thick contents" or complicated cysts, which show internal echoes in B mode, whereas in harmonic mode they appear anechoic [20] (fig. 11).

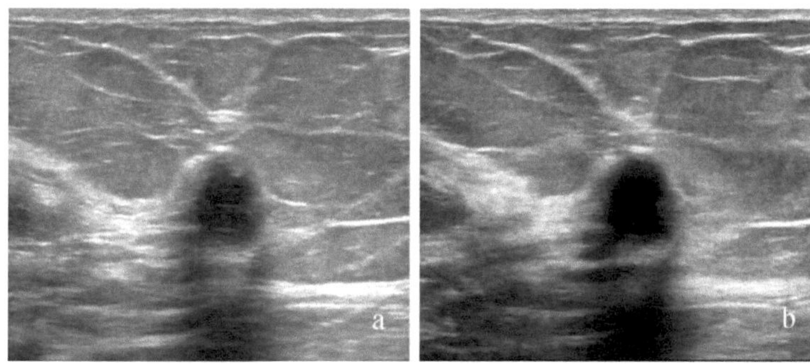

Fig. 11: Harmonic mode (a) B-mode ultrasound. Hypoechoic mass, (b) Harmonic mode ultrasound. Cystic anechogenic mass with thickened wall. Histology. Histology: reworked cyst.

2.3. Composite mode (Compound)

D two types of composite, frequency composite (several different ultrasound emission frequencies are used to reconstruct the final image), and spatial composite (several ultrasound emission angles are used and combined into a single composite image). This technique limits artifacts, improves analysis of lesion contours, better defines the internal echostructure of masses and enables detection of small lesions [21] (fig. 12). It also enables better detection of intra-lesional calcifications [22]. On the other hand, posterior ultrasound changes are attenuated [23].

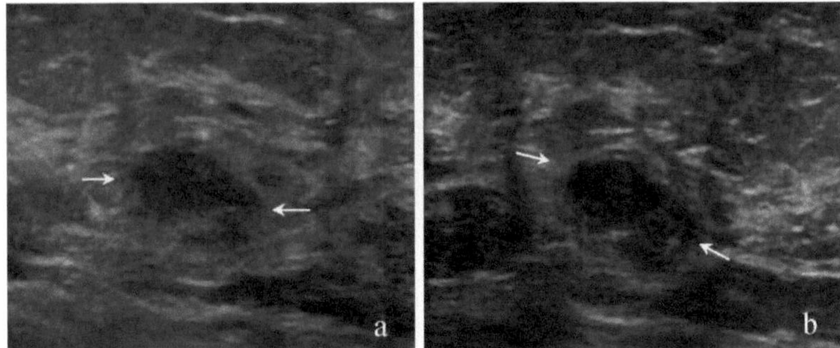

Fig. 12. Composite mode. (a) B-mode ultrasound. Hypoechoic mass with indistinct contours, (b) Composite-mode ultrasound. Hypoechoic, circumscribed mass. Histology: Adenofibroma.

2.4. Doppler mode

It detects tumor angiogenesis. Malignant lesions are generally more vascularized than benign ones, with an abnormal, irregular appearance of the vessels. Detection and spectrum analysis of these vessels require a probe of at least 10 MHz and a rigorous ultrasound technique (adjustment of focus, reduction of overall gain, adaptation of the size of the Doppler box, filtering to the minimum 10 in order to analyze low frequencies, no pressure on the breast to avoid obliteration of small vessels) [24, 25].

Energy Doppler has better sensitivity to slow flows, but is more sensitive to artifacts [34]. Doppler can be used to analyze hypoechoic lesions of a "cystic or solid" nature. The presence of vascularization in an echogenic lesion indicates that the lesion is tissue-based. On the other hand, the absence of vascularization does not rule out the presence of a tissue portion [15] (fig. 13).

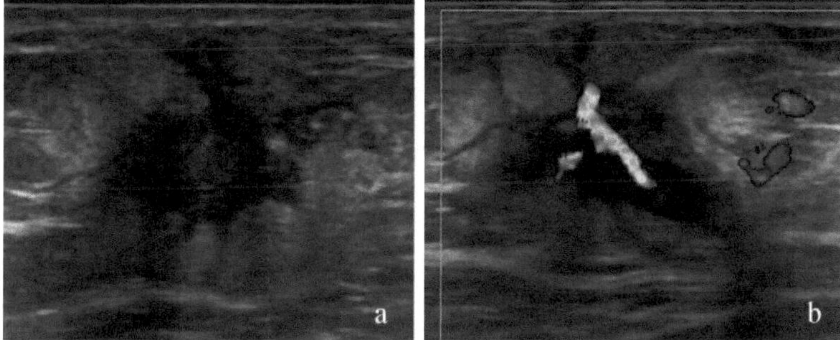

Fig. 13: Doppler mode (a) B-mode ultrasound. Hypoechoic mass with spiculated contours, (b) Doppler mode ultrasound. Intralesional vascularization.

2.5 Elastography

Elastography is a non-invasive technique used in conjunction with ultrasound to qualitatively, semi-quantitatively or quantitatively assess the deformability of lesions subjected to stress [26, 27]. The image obtained is then translated into an elastogram. This technique was developed to improve the specificity of B-mode breast ultrasound, by adding compressibility and lesion "hardness" to the criteria of echostructure and lesion morphology (fig. 14). Breast elastography uses two distinct modes: free-hand elastography and shear-wave elastography.

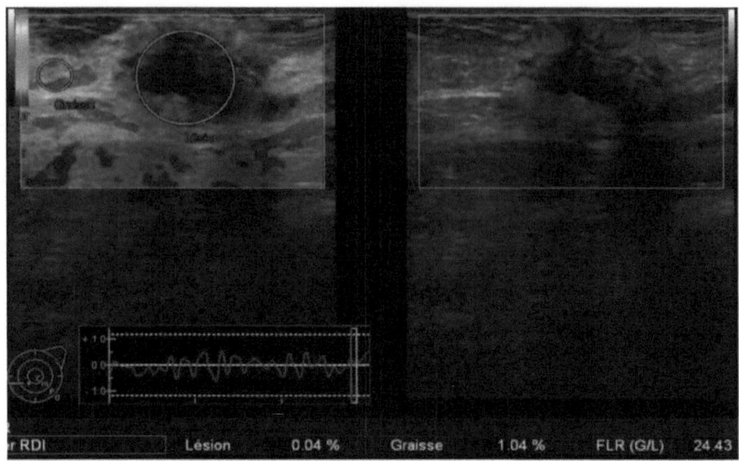

Fig. 14. Elastography. Elastography. Calculation of elasticity ratio in standard deviation.

3. Breast MRI

3.1 Equipment

3.1.1 Magnetic field

Magnetic field strength influences acquisition time and image quality. The higher the magnetic field intensity, the better the image resolution and the shorter the sequence time. Most teams work with magnetic fields of 1.5 tesla (T).

3.1.2 Antennas

Breast MRI must be performed using dedicated breast antennas that follow the shape of the breasts (fig. 15). The use of parallel imaging improves the performance of these antennas, increasing surface coverage, signal uniformity and temporal and spatial resolution [28]. The breasts must be well positioned in the antenna, with the nipple at the zenith, integrating the whole breast into the antenna and avoiding folds (fig. 16).

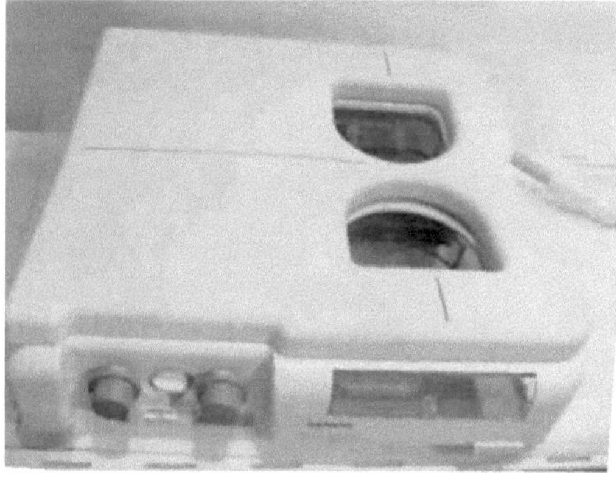

Fig. 15. Antenna breast.

The breast should not be overly compressed. Compression serves to wedge the breasts to prevent their movement in the antenna. Excessive compression of the breast can falsely reduce the size of lesions, thus changing the TNM classification [29]. Compression can also reduce the amplitude of enhancement and alter the enhancement curve (fig. 17).

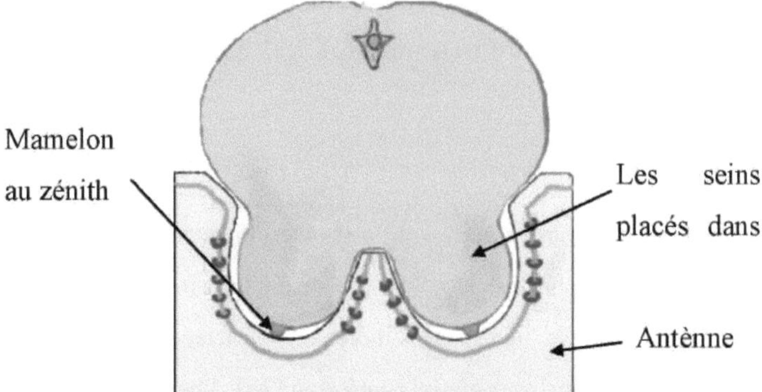

Fig. 16. Position of breasts in the anterior.

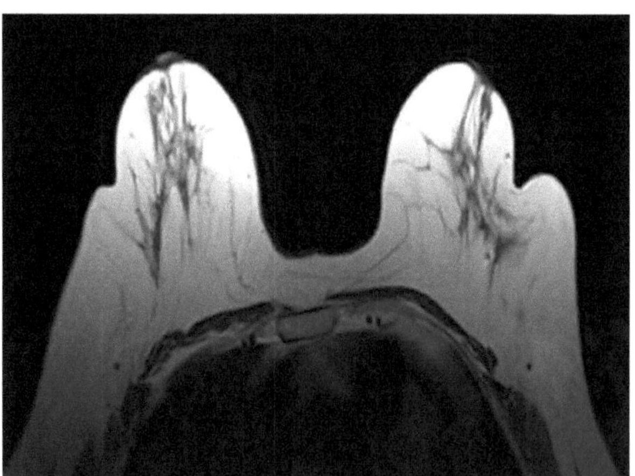

Fig. 17. Compression defect. T2-weighted sequence.

3.2 Time of examination

The timing of the examination is essential for the best interpretation of breast MRI. Avoid the second half of the cycle, when physiological glandular enhancement is most marked. It is minimal in the 2nd week of the menstrual cycle in patients with genital activity. Outside this period, non-specific diffuse or focal contrast enhancement may be present, leading to misinterpretation (fig. 18). Glandular enhancement is increased by hormone replacement therapy in post-menopausal women, with up to 50% of women showing non-specific enhancement. In the event of an uninterpretable examination in post-menopausal women, the test should be discontinued for 3 months.

For post-operative MRI, a minimum delay of one month must be observed to limit enhancement secondary to inflammatory phenomena. The optimum time for performing breast MRI is at least six months after the end of treatment [3032].

Percutaneous microbiopsies generally have no impact on the interpretation of contrast-enhanced MRI. However, the topography, date of biopsy and results, if available, should always be mentioned. Oral contraception also has no impact on the use of breast MRI.

3.3 Installing the patient

A venous access with long tubing is set up. The patient is then placed in procubitus position, with her arms over her head as comfortably as possible, to ensure the immobility required for the examination. The breasts placed in the antenna must be well supported; if necessary, a foam pad can be used to prevent small breasts from moving in the antenna.

3.4 Injection of contrast media

Breast MRI highlights intratumoral neoangiogenesis through contrast injection, enabling lesions to be detected [33]. The contrast medium used is gadolinium chelate. The injected dose is 0.1 mmol/kg body weight. The injection rate should be 2 to 3 ml per second. Injection of the contrast medium is followed by an injection of 20 ml of saline at the same flow rate, to avoid stagnation of the contrast medium in the tubing.

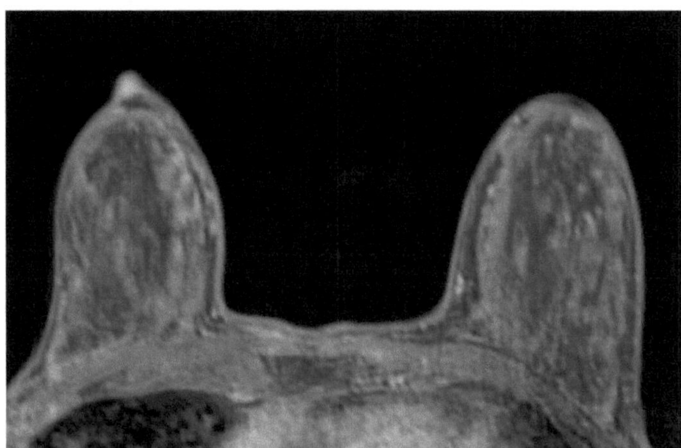

Fig. 18. Physiological glandular enhancement. Subtracted sequence injected.

3.5 Breast MRI protocols

3.5.1 Acquisition plan

Fields of view must be sufficiently wide to allow analysis of both breasts, both nipple-areolar plates (NAPs), the axillary hollows and the chest wall [33, 34].

Acquisition in the axial plane is the most frequently used. This acquisition plane enables dynamic sequences of the breasts to be performed in 1 minute. The advantages of the axial plane are comparative analysis of the whole of both breasts, which facilitates detection of abnormal contrast, and analysis of the PAMs, axillary recesses and chest wall [34]. Cardiorespiratory artifacts degrade acquisition quality. Phase encoding from right to left instead of anteroposterior reduces these artifacts.

Acquisition in the sagittal plane reduces the field of view. This in turn improves image resolution and the quality of fat suppression techniques [33]. Finally, sagittal acquisition also enables better analysis of physiological glandular enhancement, which facilitates anatomical study. Nevertheless, the study of both breasts, including the axillary hollows, requires a large number of slices, which prolongs examination time [34].

Coronal acquisition reduces cardiac artifacts. But this plane is often degraded by respiratory and flow artifacts. This acquisition plane also requires many slices to be able to analyze the entire breast from the chest wall to the PAM [34].

3.5.2 Cutting thickness

Slice thickness must be thin, less than or equal to 3 mm, with pixel and voxel sizes of less than 1 mm. To enable us to carry out multiplanar reconstructions.

3.5.3 Breast MRI sequences

3.5.3.1 Morphological sequences

In the past, uninjected T2- and T1-weighted sequences in breast MRI were not considered very useful, due to their low diagnostic value. Since then, many authors have demonstrated the value of using morphological sequences.

T2-weighted sequences can be used to detect cystic lesions whose presence indicates benign enhancement, whether annular enhancement in inflammatory cysts or non-mass enhancement in fibrocystic mastopathy.

T2-weighted sequences with fat saturation are very useful in the case of nipple discharge, enabling indirect MRI galactography images to be created, and also improve the detection of small cancers (fig. 19).

T1-weighted sequences without fat saturation are useful for detecting the presence of a fatty component in a lesion, an important factor in favor of benignity (fig. 20). These sequences are also useful for confirming the correct position of metal markers in the biopsy site [35] (fig. 21).

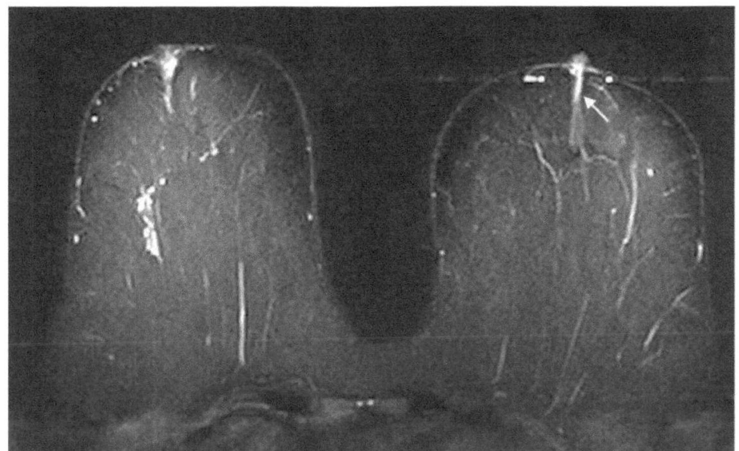

Fig. 19. Ductal ectasia. Intracanal hypersignal on T2 sequences with fat supression (arrows).

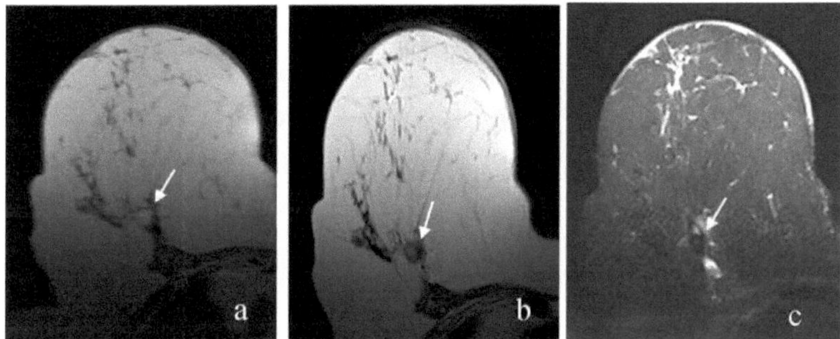

Fig. 20. Cytosteatonecrosis: (a) T1 sequence, (b) T2 sequence, (c) T2 Fat Sat sequence. Lesion hypersignal T1, hypersignal T2, hyposignal on T2 sequence with fat supression (arrows).

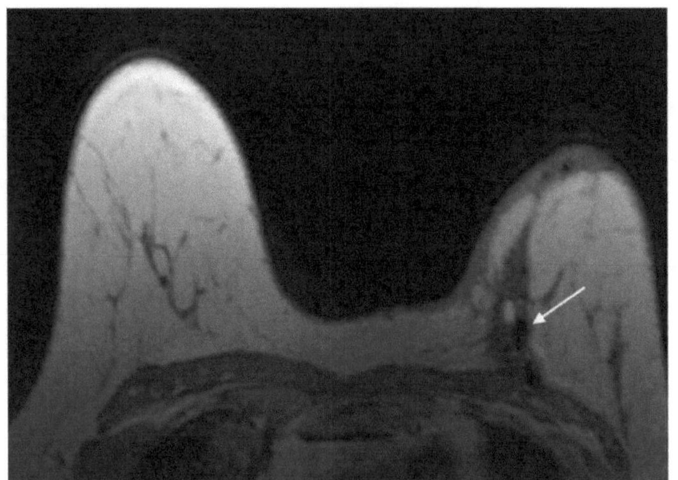

Fig. 21. Position of metal marker in ground on T1 sequence (arrow).

3.5.3.2 Dynamic sequences

Dynamic analysis makes it possible to distinguish suspicious abnormal angiogenesis among the various enhancement kinetics. T1 gradient echo sequences after injection of gadolinium chelate (fig. 22).

2D or 3D acquisition?

Compared with 2D sequences, 3D sequences give finer slices with a better signal-to-noise ratio [32]. On the other hand, as 3D acquisition is performed without fat suppression, it is desirable to use 2D sequences to reduce phase-encoding artifacts that extend in all three directions in 3D sequences, masking contours and making it difficult to detect these artifacts on subtraction sequences.

The 3D sequence enables volume analysis of the lesion (measurement in 3 planes, distance from the nipple-areolar plate and the deep pectoral plane) (fig. 23).

3.5.3.3 Complementary sequences

- **Broadcast**

The principle of diffusion imaging is to quantify the movement of water molecules in tissues. The objectives of diffusion sequences are to optimize detection of small lesions and improve characterization of benign and malignant lesions. Diffusion MRI can also be used to assess the response to neoadjuvant chemotherapy. An increase of more than 10% in ADC coefficients at the end of the first cycle of chemotherapy signifies a decrease in cell density, and is therefore predictive of response to treatment [36, 37].

- **Magnetic resonance spectroscopy**

Spectroscopy is a molecular imaging technique. Its principle is to highlight an abnormal choline peak in malignant tumors (resonance at 3.2 ppm) [38]. Bartella et al. reported that the addition of spectroscopy to the standard protocol improved the PPV of biopsies from 35% to 82% ($p < 0.01$), and enabled biopsy to be avoided in 57% of lesions [39]. In addition, numerous studies have shown that this sequence enables early response (at 24 h) to neoadjuvant chemotherapy to be demonstrated [40].

The three types of spectroscopic enhancement curves described by CK. Kuhl et al [41]:

- Type I: an initial slow, then progressive enhancement curve (fig. 24)
- Type II: a rapid initial enhancement curve, followed by a plateau (fig. 25).
- Type III: a rapid initial enhancement curve, followed by a washout (fig. 26).

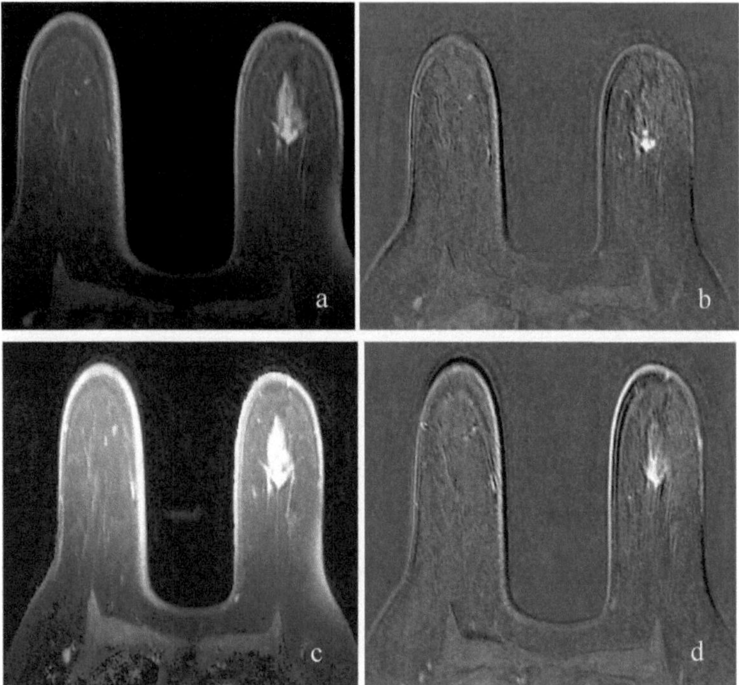

Fig. 22. Enhancement analysis of a malignant tumor of the left breast. Dynamic analysis enables the tumor to be distinguished from the rest of the fibroglandular parenchyma thanks to acquisition before the second minute in three-dimensional (3D) T1 weighting (a) and 3D T1 injected with subtraction (b). At six minutes, it is difficult to differentiate the cancer from the breast parenchyma on T1 3D injected (c) and T1 3D injected with subtraction (d) sequences.

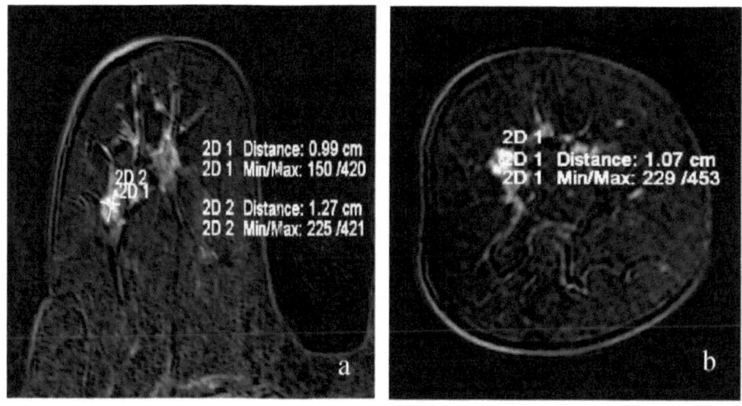

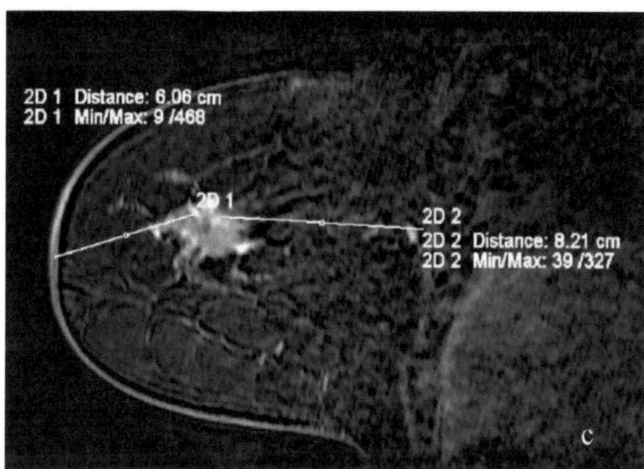

Fig. 23. Injected 3D T1-weighted sequence with subtraction. Analysis of lesion volume (measurement in 3 planes (a + b), lesion distance from the nipple-areolar plate and the deep pectoral plane (c).

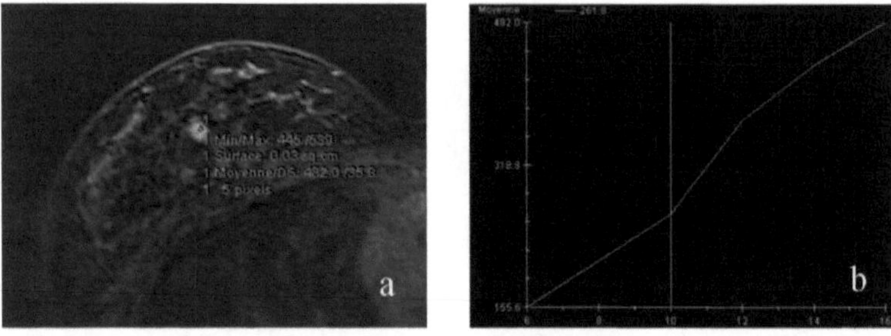

Fig. 24. Type I curve. (a) Subtracted injected sequences, axial section. (b) Enhancement curve. Histology: fibroadenoma.

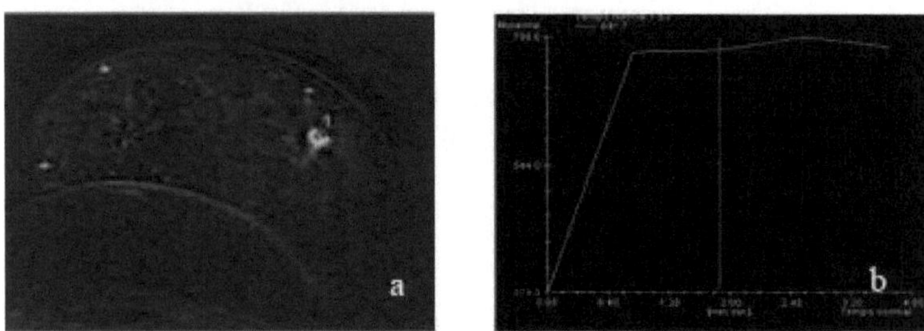

Fig. 25: Type II curve (a) Subtracted injected sequences, axial section. (b) Enhancement curve. Histology: fibroadenoma.

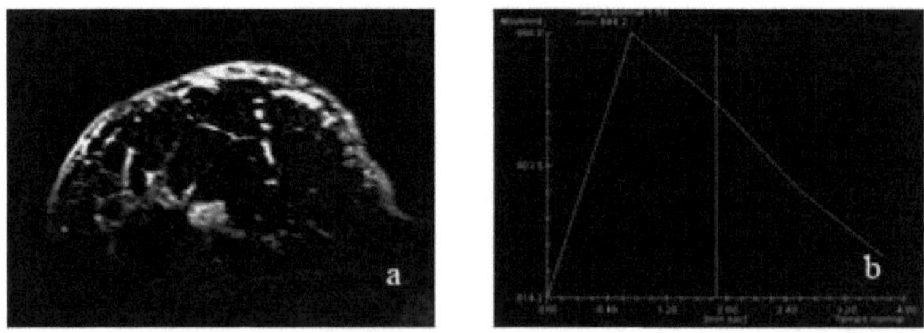

Fig. 26. type III curve: (a) Subtracted injected sequences, axial section. (b) Enhancement curve. Histology: Invasive lobular carcinoma.

Malignant tumors

1. Ductal carcinoma in situ (DCIS)

Ductal cancers in situ represent a heterogeneous group of lesions corresponding to the proliferation of cohesive cells in the lumen of acini and ducts, while respecting the myo-epithelial cell layer and basement membrane. With the advent of screening, 80-85% of ductal cancers in situ are diagnosed at the subclinical stage [42].

1.1. Epidemiology

Intracanal carcinoma of the breast is the precursor of invasive carcinoma. It accounts for between 15% and 20% of cancers detected [43]. Incidence also varies according to the histological type of IBCC. The incidence of CCIS with comedo-necrosis has increased by 15 to 22 times, while the incidence of lesions without comedo-necrosis has remained stable [44].

Incidence varies with age. It rises progressively, peaking between the ages of 65 and 69, then declines until the age of 79.

1.2. Clinic

They may manifest as a palpable mass, a clear or bloody uniparous nipple discharge, or more rarely, Paget's disease of the nipple. The diagnosis may be made incidentally during analysis of a surgical biopsy for breast reduction.

1.3. Histology

Ductal carcinomas in situ are classified according to three criteria: the architecture of proliferation, the degree of cytonuclear atypia and the presence or absence of tumour necrosis, sometimes calcified (fig. 27).

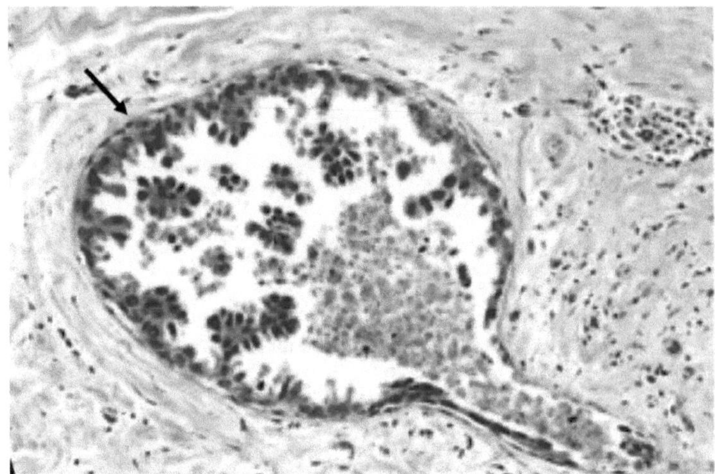

Fig. 27. Ductal carcinoma in situ. Histology. Epithelial tumour proliferation not extending beyond the basement membrane (arrow) [45].

1.4. Imaging

On mammography, carcinoma in situ is manifested in 80% of cases by a focus of calcifications (figs. 28, 29, 30). Calcifications are either secretory in origin, of unsuspicious morphology, round and powdery in 57% of cases, or cellular necrosis, essentially irregular, vermicular punctiform microcalcifications [42, 46-48]. The shape and distribution of calcifications, such as non-round focus, segmental or linear distribution, are most often elements in favor of CCIS.

Other mammographic abnormalities are much less frequent. In less than 10% of cases, there may be an irregularly shaped mass, or architectural distortion in less than 10% of cases.

Ultrasound is used in conjunction with this, to detect a homogeneous hypoechoic mass with microlobulated contours, which may or may not be associated with calcifications and which is not very suspicious in appearance [49] (fig. 30).

On elastography, a number of previous studies have shown that carcinomas in situ tend to be less hard than infiltrating carcinomas [5056]. Bae JS et al [52] compared 70 ductal carcinomas in situ against 50 infiltrating carcinomas of the nonspecific type and found lower elasticity values for ductal carcinomas in situ than for infiltrating carcinomas of the nonspecific type, 74.8 ± 47.4 kPa vs. 118.71 ± 70.5 kPa respectively, $p < 0.0001$. Shin J et al [53] also reported lower elasticity values in ductal carcinomas in situ than in non-specific infiltrating carcinomas (85.33 ± 66.1 kPa vs. 119.04 ± 73.32 kPa, $p = 0.041$). The hardness of infiltrating carcinomas is high (Fig. 30). This is partly due to the extracellular fibrous matrix produced by fibroblasts [57].

On MRI, non-mass enhancement is often found in patients with CCIS lesions, ranging from 60% to 81% depending on the series [58, 59] (fig. 31).

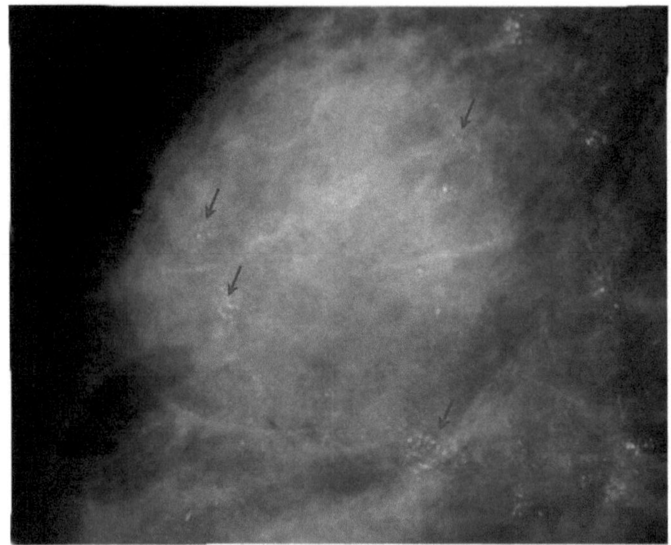

Fig. 28. Ductal carcinoma in situ. Mammogram. Multiple foci of amorphous, polymorphous microcalcifications (arrows).

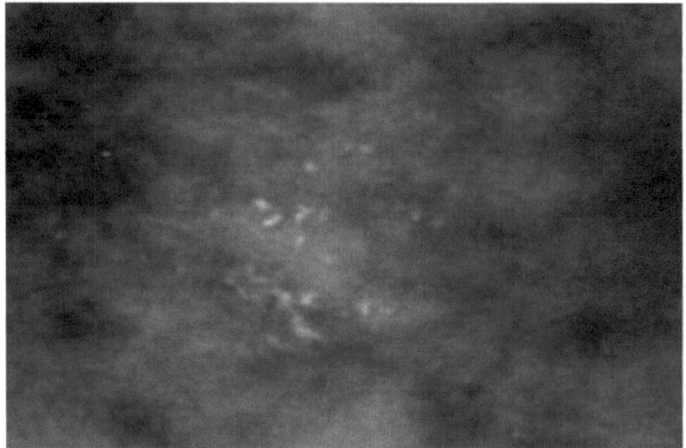

Fig. 29. Ductal comedocarcinoma in situ. Mammogram. Focal point of polymorphous microcalcifications.

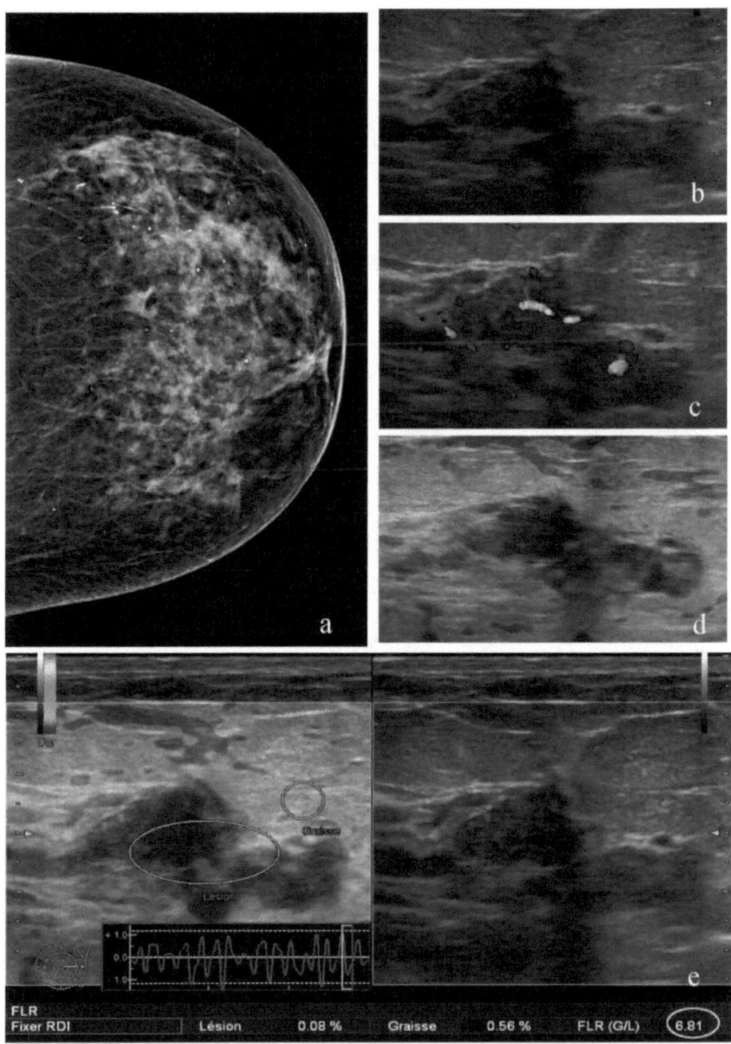

Fig. 30. Ductal carcinoma in situ. (a) Mammography. Mixed breast density, conjunctivo-grandular and fatty. Absence of mass. Macrocalcifications (arrows). (b) B-mode ultrasound. Irregularly shaped mass with microlobulated contours, fine interface, no posterior acoustic effect. (c) Color Doppler. Hypervascularized mass. (d+e) Elastography. Hard lesion, graded 4 with an elasticity ratio of 6.81.

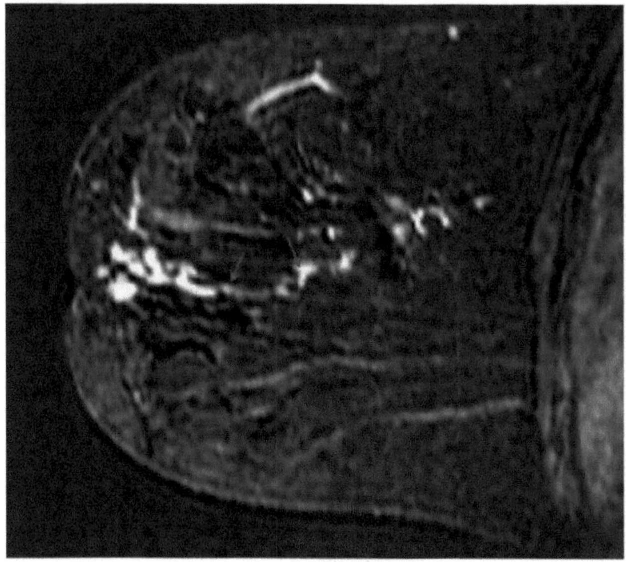

Fig. 31. Ductal carcinoma in situ. MRI SCAN. Injected Tl Fat Sat sequence.

Linear non-mass enhancement converging towards the nipple.

2. Lobular carcinoma in situ (CLIS)

Lobular carcinoma in situ is characterized by a proliferation of small, loosely cohesive cells with regular, rounded nuclei in the breast lobules. Multiple or bilateral localization is common.

2.1 Epidemiology

CLIS represent around 10-15% of in situ breast cancers and 0.7% of lobular carcinomas [60-63]. The average age of onset of CLIS is in the forties, and almost two-thirds are in the premenopausal phase [64-66]. Its frequency varies between 0.8% and 3.8% [67, 68], and it is found in 0.8% to 2% of biopsies taken for benign lesions [68].

2.2 Histology

According to the WHO, CLIS is defined as a carcinoma involving the intralobular canaliculi without invasion of neighboring connective tissue. It is considered a risk factor for invasive cancer rather than a cancerous condition [3].

2.3 Imaging

They have no specific radiological translation and are discovered incidentally during histological analysis of associated benign lesions. CLIS are mainly seen as microcalcifications, in around 95% of cases, rarely as a round mass or architectural disorganization (fig. 32).

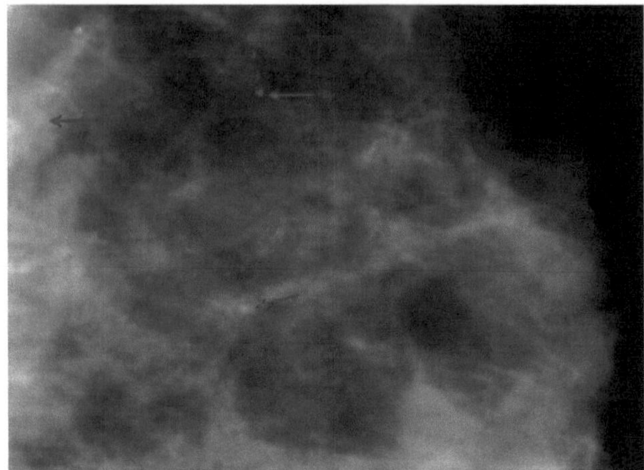

Fig. 32. lobular carcinoma in situ. Mammogram. Irregular, polymorphic microcalcifications, few in number (arrows) [69].

3. Non-specific infiltrating carcinoma (NSIAC)

CINST is defined by a proliferation of ductal epithelial cells that cross the basement membrane, infiltrating the breast tissue where lymphatic and blood vessels are located. It is the most common histological type of breast cancer. It accounts for 70-80% of infiltrating cancers [70].

3.1 Clinic

It most often manifests as a palpable mass. With the advent of screening, diagnosis of CINST at sub-clinical stage is on the increase.

3.2 Histology

Macroscopically, it is a hard tumor with star-shaped outlines, rarely soft or with sharp outlines [71]. Microscopically, the appearance varies greatly according to the degree of differentiation and the ability of the tumour cells to form tubes, trabeculae or masses (fig. 33).

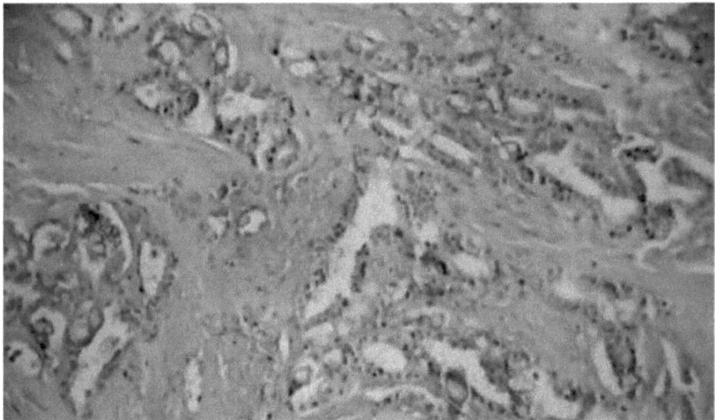

Fig. 33. CINST. Microscopy. Destruction of normal epithelial structures by infiltrating malignant proliferation.

3.3 Imaging

The imaging aspects are well known, most often in the form of an irregular or stellate mass, architectural distortion, microcalcifications, rarely a round mass [72].

On mammography, CINST classically presents as a hyperdense, spiculated mass (figs. 34, 35). Rarely, it may appear as a circumscribed mass (fig. 36).

On ultrasonography, it appears as an irregularly shaped, spiculated, hypoechoic, attenuating mass with a long axis not parallel to the skin, surrounded by haloechogenesis (figs. 37, 38). More rarely, it presents as a circumscribed mass with posterior enhancement (fig. 39).

Elastography confirms the diagnosis of a lesion suspected of malignancy, showing high hardness compared with adjacent breast tissue (fig. 40, 41).

MRI, in turn, shows a classic mass suspicious of malignancy, i.e. an irregular, spiculated mass with heterogeneous enhancement, sometimes annular (figs. 42, 43, 44).

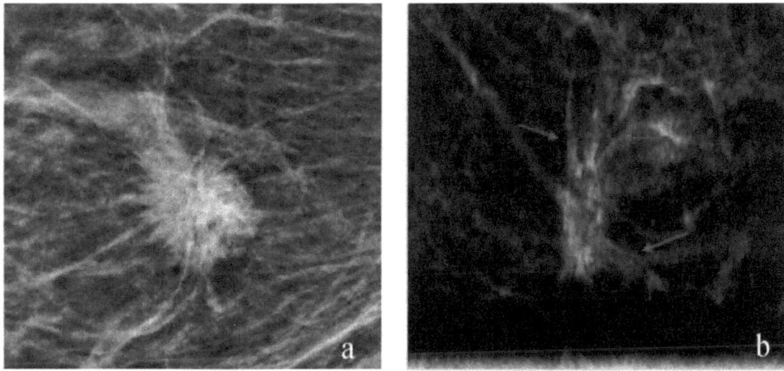

Fig. 34. CINST. Mammogram. (a) Mass in a 45-year-old woman. (b) Mass in a 58-year-old woman. Hyperdense, irregularly shaped mass with spiculated contours (arrows).

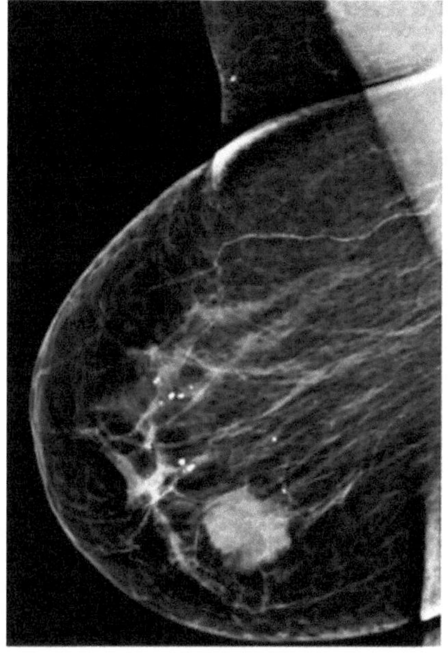

Fig. 35. CINST in a 71-year-old woman. Mammogram. Hyperdense, irregularly shaped mass with irregular contours (arrow).

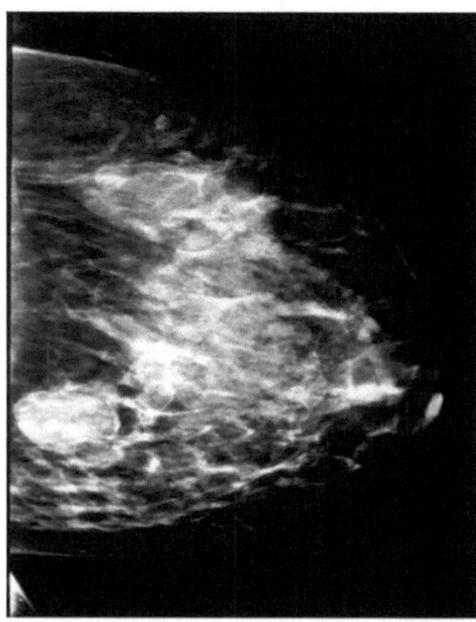

Fig. 36. CINST in a 43-year-old woman. Mammogram. Hyperdense, round mass with circumscribed contours (arrow).

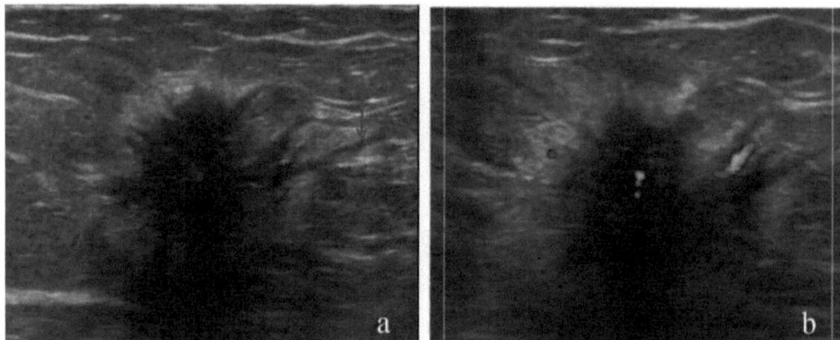

Fig. 37. CINST in a 45-year-old woman. (a) B-mode ultrasonography. Irregularly shaped mass with spiculated (arrow-shaped) contours, hypoechoic with posterior attenuation, surrounded by a peripheral echogenic halo. (b) Color Doppler. Mass with peripheral and central vascularization.

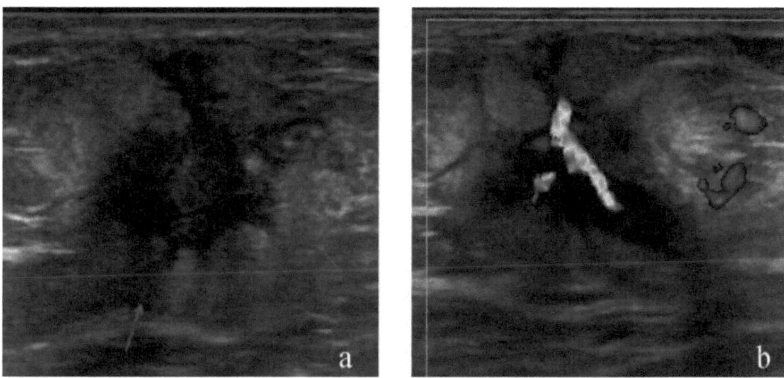

Fig. 38. CINST in a 52-year-old woman. (a) B-mode ultrasound. Irregularly shaped mass with spiculated contours (arrows), hypoechoic, surrounded by a prominent peripheral echogenic halo. (b) Color Doppler. Mass with peripheral and central vascularization.

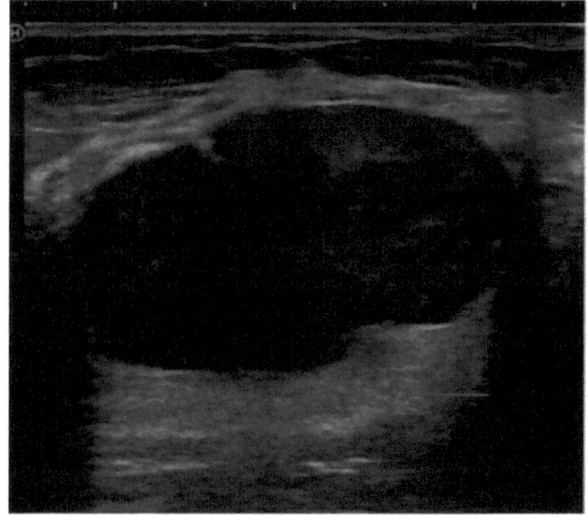

Fig. 39. CINST in a 49-year-old woman. B-mode ultrasonography. Oval-shaped mass, lobulated contours, strongly hypoechoic, abrupt interface with posterior enhancement (arrow).

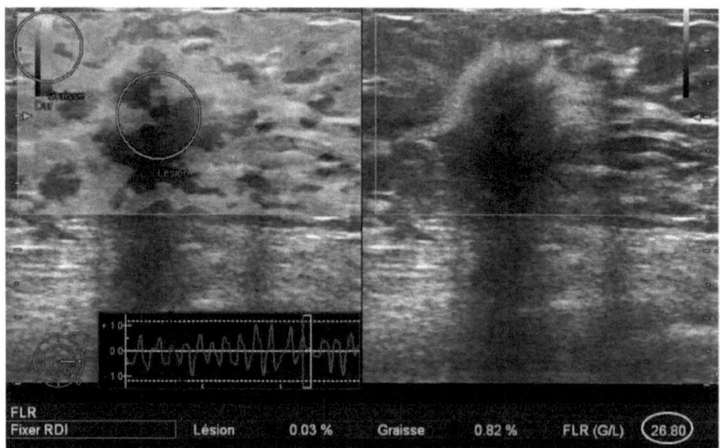

Fig. 40. CINST in a 45-year-old woman. Elastography. Hard mass with an elasticity ratio of 26.80.

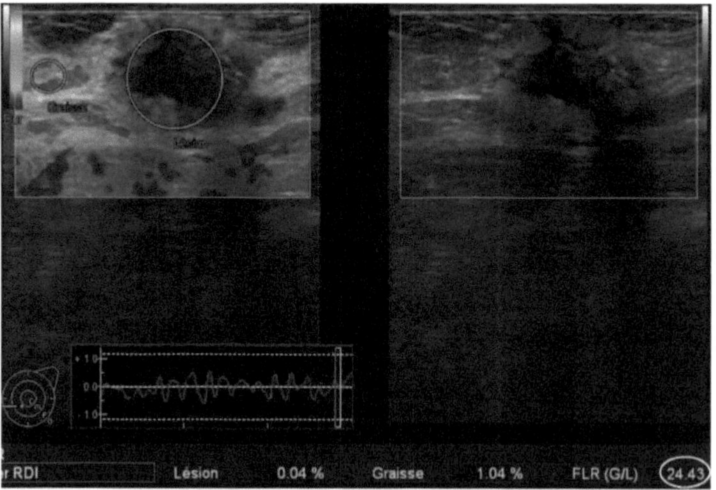

Fig. 41. CINST in a 52-year-old woman. Elastography. Hard lesion, graded 5 with an elasticity ratio of 24.43.

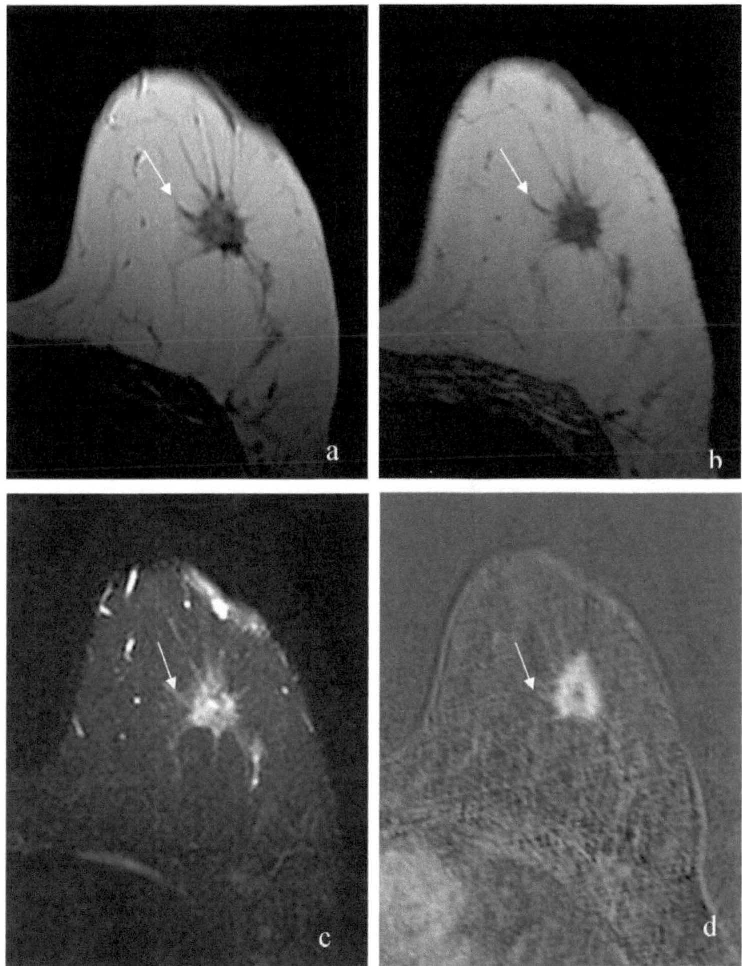

Fig. 42. CINST (a) T2-weighted sequence, (b) T1-weighted sequence, (c) T2 Fat Sat sequence, (d) injected subtraction sequence. Irregular mass with spiculated contours, hyposignal T1 and T2, hypersignal T2 Fat Sat, heterogeneous enhancement on injected subtraction sequences with presence of spicules (arrows).

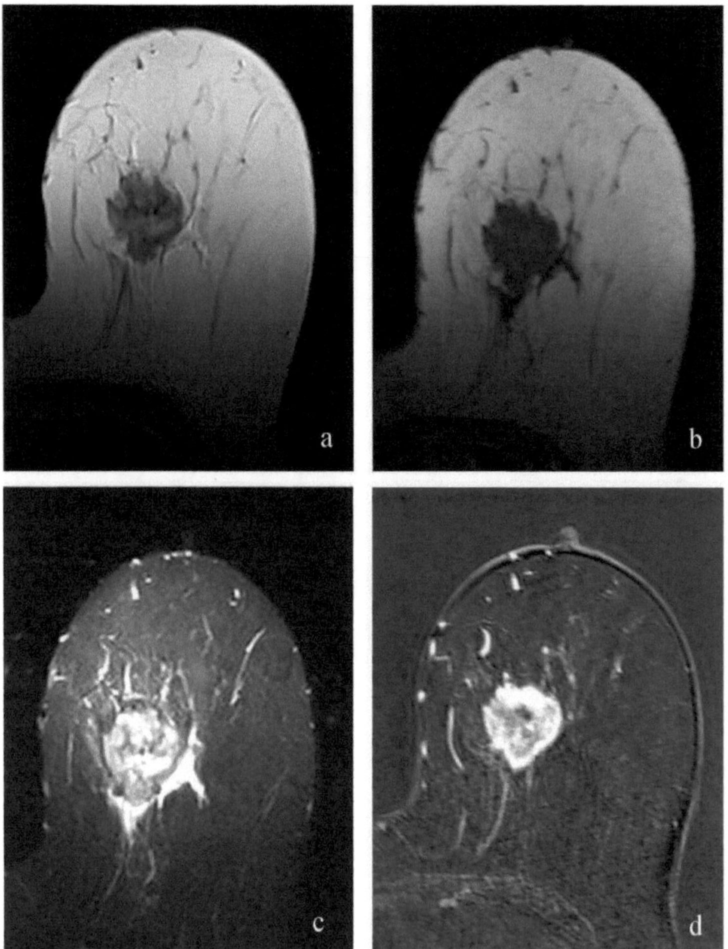

Fig. 43. CINST (a) T2-weighted sequence, (b) T1-weighted sequence, (c) T2 Fat Sat sequence, (d) injected subtraction sequence. Irregular mass with irregular contours, hyposignal T1 and T2, hyposignal T2 Fat Sat, heterogeneous enhancement on injected subtraction sequences (arrow).

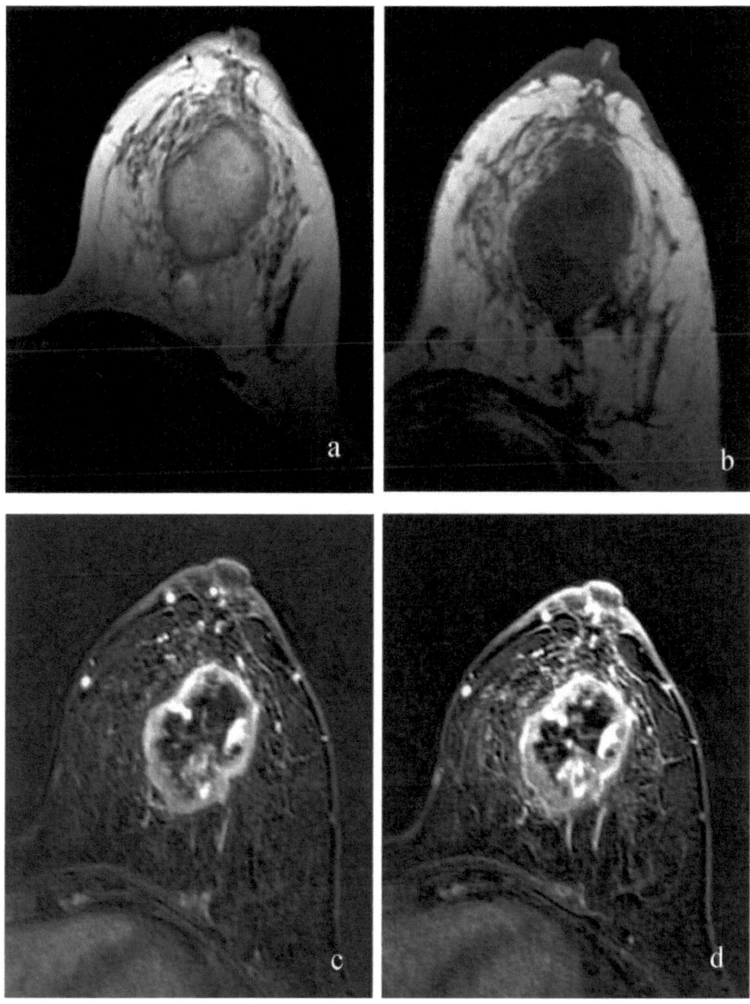

Fig. 44. CINST. (a) T2-weighted sequence. (b) T-weighted sequence. (c) Native injected T1 sequence. (d) Injected subtracted sequence. Irregularly shaped and contoured mass, hyposignal T1, hypersignal T2, annular enhancement on injected sequences (arrows).

4. Invasive lobular carcinoma

Infiltrating lobular carcinoma is the second most common histological type after non-specific infiltrating carcinoma [73]. It accounts for around 10-15% of all infiltrating breast cancers [73, 74]. The incidence of infiltrating lobular carcinoma is rising sharply, mainly in post-menopausal women [75].

4.1. Histology

Macroscopically, they are often irregular, poorly circumscribed masses that are difficult to measure. Microscopically, infiltrating lobular carcinomas are made up of small, round, non-cohesive cells, isolated or in "Indian file", tending to infiltrate adjacent breast tissue, without destroying anatomical structures or causing a frank desmoplastic reaction [76] (fig. 45).

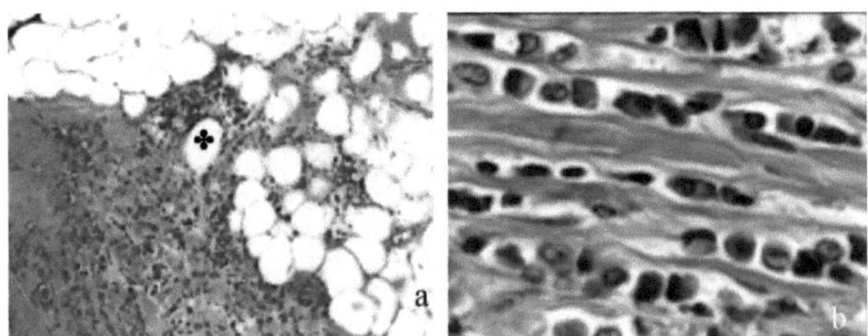

Fig. 45. Invasive lobular carcinoma. Microscopy. (a) Infiltration of fatty tissue by isolated cells without fibrous reaction stroma (asterisk). (b) "Indian file" arrangement of cells [77].

4.2 Imaging

The originality of infiltrating lobular carcinoma in imaging lies mainly in the difficulty of detecting it on mammography and breast ultrasound. It can have particular and sometimes subtle presentations [78, 79]. It is the main cause of false-negative and interval cancers [80-82]. The second difficulty with infiltrating lobular carcinoma is the assessment of its size. It is particularly difficult to assess the extent of lesions on mammography and breast ultrasound, and preoperative MRI is usually indicated [83-86].

On mammography, infiltrating lobular carcinomas often present as subtle images, such as a sparse mass, asymmetry and architectural distortion, often visible only on a single incidence and rarely associated with microcalcifications (fig. 46).

On ultrasonography, the most frequently observed abnormality is an irregular hypoechoic mass [87] (fig. 47). Occasionally, infiltrating lobular carcinomas may present as an isolated posterior shadow cone with no identifiable mass (fig. 48) [78]. They less often have a long vertical axis and are more frequently hyperechoic or with a hyperechoic portion [79, 88, 89]. However, there are still cases where ultrasound shows no abnormality [90].

In studies by Aoudia et al [91], 30 infiltrating lobular carcinomas were compared with 55 non-specific infiltrating carcinomas. The infiltrating lobular carcinomas were harder than the non-specific infiltrating carcinomas, with a mean elasticity ratio of 56.4 ± 46.28 and 28.43 ± 35.43 respectively, with a significant difference (P = 0.004) (fig. 49). Similarly, Brkljacic et al [92], infiltrating lobular carcinomas had a higher mean elasticity ratio than non-specific infiltrating carcinomas, 180.41 + 27.06 kPa vs. 162.20 + 37.46

kPa respectively, $P < 0.05$.

Elastography seems to better reflect the extent of lesions compared with B-mode ultrasonography. In the study by Aoudia et al [91], infiltrating lobular carcinomas had higher size ratio values than non-specific infiltrating carcinomas, respectively 1.56 ± 0.39 and 1.21 ± 0.14 ($P < 0.001$) (fig. 47, 48). This is explained by the particular histological nature of infiltrating lobular carcinomas, which are made up of small, round, non-cohesive cells, isolated or in "Indian file", tending to infiltrate adjacent breast tissue without destroying it [93].

MRI is widely recognized as the most sensitive detection modality for infiltrating lobular carcinoma, with a sensitivity of 83% to 100% [94-99]. This sensitivity is superior to that of other diagnostic modalities, ranging from 65% to 98% for clinical examination, 81% to 98% for mammography and 68% to 98% for ultrasound [80, 82, 83, 88, 100]. Most lesions present as mass-like enhancements of irregular or even spiculated shape and contour [101] (fig. 50). Other MRI abnormalities may be seen, such as a main mass surrounded by multiple foci, or focal, regional, multifocal heterogeneous non-mass enhancement, or septal contrast without a dominant mass (fig. 51).

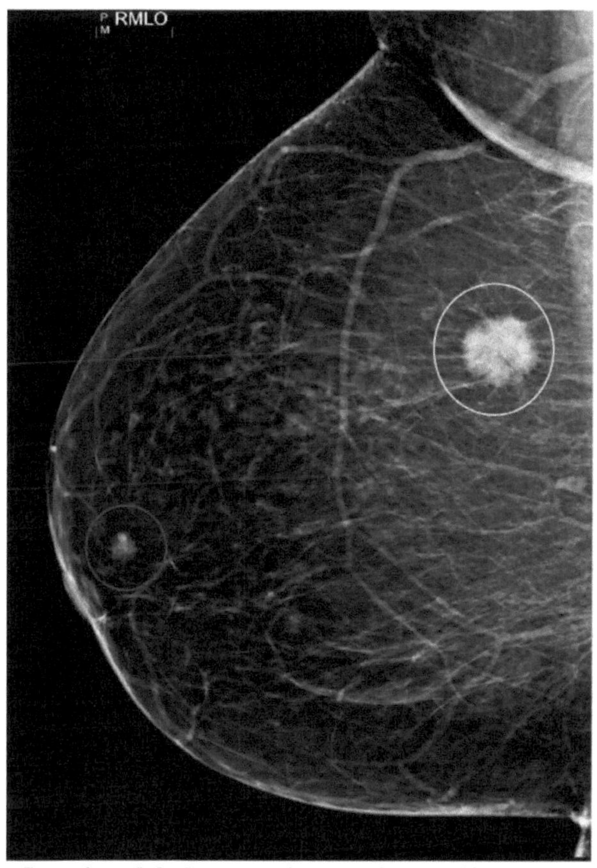

Fig. 46. Invasive lobular carcinoma in a 48-year-old woman. Mammogram. Small, sparse retroareolar mass with irregular contours (red circle). Histology: infiltrating lobular carcinoma. Associated with another hyperdense, spiculated mass (yellow circle). Histology: CINST.

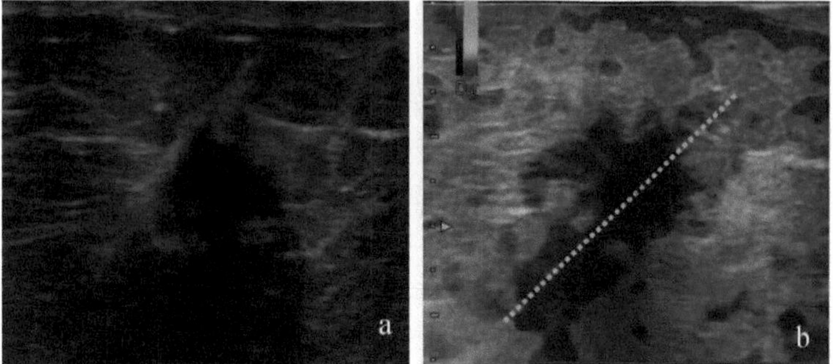

Fig. 47. Invasive lobular carcinoma in a 48-year-old woman. (a) B-mode ultrasonography. Irregularly shaped mass with spiculated contours and thin interface with posterior attenuation. (b) Elastography. Hard mass, appears more extensive than in B-mode.

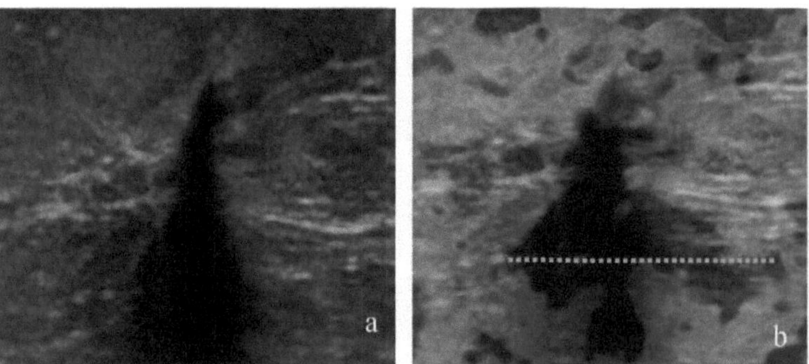

Fig. 48. Invasive lobular carcinoma in a 50-year-old woman (a) B-mode ultrasound. Ultrasound beam attenuation, no clearly visible mass. (b) Elastography. Attenuating lesion in B-mode is better visible and more extensive on elastography.

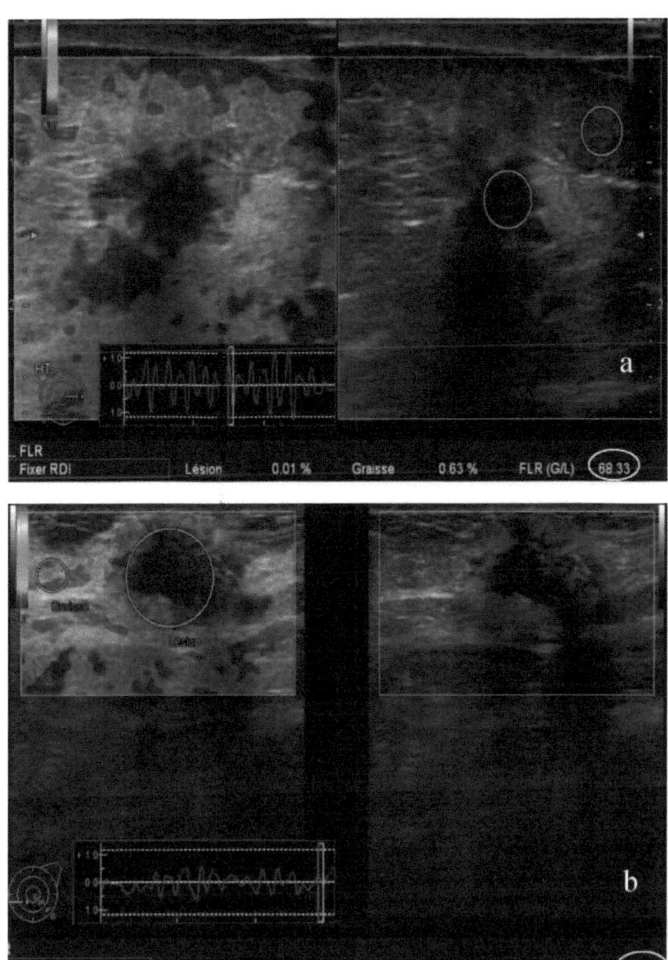

Fig. 49. Invasive lobular carcinoma vs. CINST. (a) Invasive lobular carcinoma (b) CINST. The mass of infiltrating lobular carcinoma is harder than CINST.

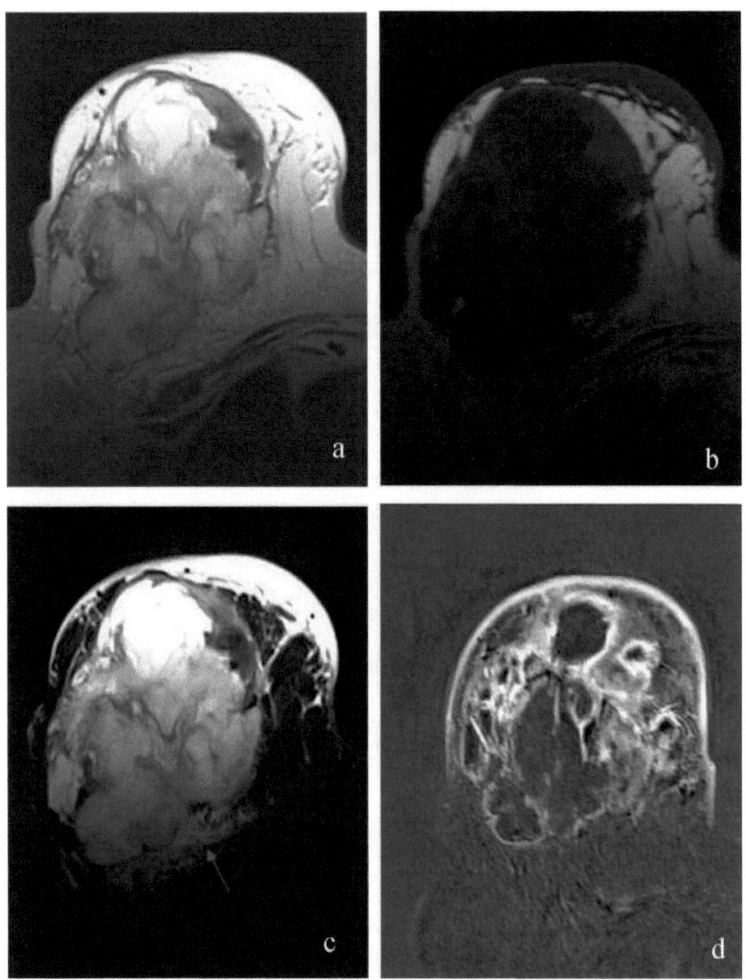

Fig. 50. Invasive lobular carcinoma (a) T2-weighted sequence (b) T1-weighted sequence (c) T2 Fat Sat sequence (c) Injected subtraction sequence. Voluminous mass with irregular shape and contours, heterogeneous T2 hypersignal, heterogeneous T1 hyposignal, annular enhancement on injected sequences.

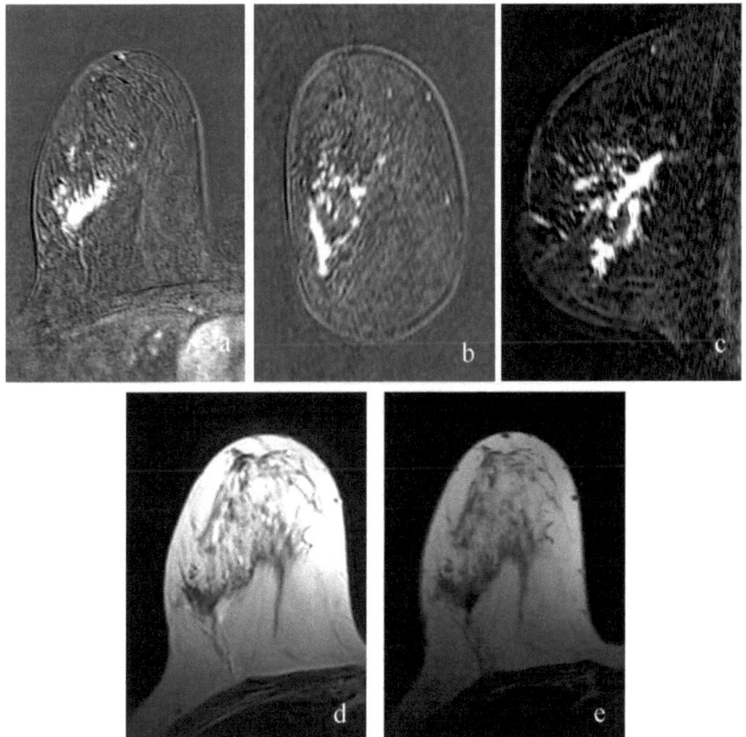

Fig. 51. Invasive lobular carcinoma (a+b+c) Injected subtraction sequences. (d) T2-weighted sequence. (e) T1-weighted sequence. Regional non-mass enhancement that does not occupy a volume in space (arrows), not visible on morphological T1 and T2 sequences.

5. Intracystic papillary carcinoma

Intracystic papillary carcinoma is a special type of breast cancer. It is a well-circumscribed epithelial tumor of the breast, with atypical papillary growth inside a dilated duct.

5.1 Epidemiology

It is a rare malignant ductal tumour, accounting for 0.5 to 1% of all breast cancers [103, 104]. It may be isolated or associated with ductal carcinoma in situ or infiltrating carcinoma [103]. The age of onset is often after 40, with a mean age ranging from 55 to 67 [104, 105]. It is characterized by slow growth and a good prognosis, with a 10-year disease-free survival rate of 91% [104, 105].

5.2 Clinic

In 50% of cases, the tumor appears as a central mass, often retroareolar. Tumor size varies between 1 and 14 cm. It may also manifest as a bloody nipple discharge, or may be discovered incidentally during a screening mammogram. Lymph node involvement is rare [103, 106].

5.3 Histology

Histologically, a thick-walled, fibrous cyst is macroscopically characterized by a nodular, rounded or poly-lobed, friable and hemorrhagic formation [104, 107]. Microscopically, the tumoral architecture is papillary, the lesion is generally localized in a cystic duct, and is characterized by a small fibrovascular arborescence devoid of a layer of myoepithelial cells, and a neoplastic epithelial proliferation presenting the morphological characteristics of a low-grade ductal carcinoma in situ [108, 109].

5.4 Imaging

Spiculated contours are rare [110, 111].

Breast ultrasonography reveals a complex cystic mass with a nodular solid component and the presence of echoes and debris in the cystic portion (Fig. 52). Color Doppler demonstrates central and peripheral vascularization of the solid portion of the mass [103, 107, 111, 112].

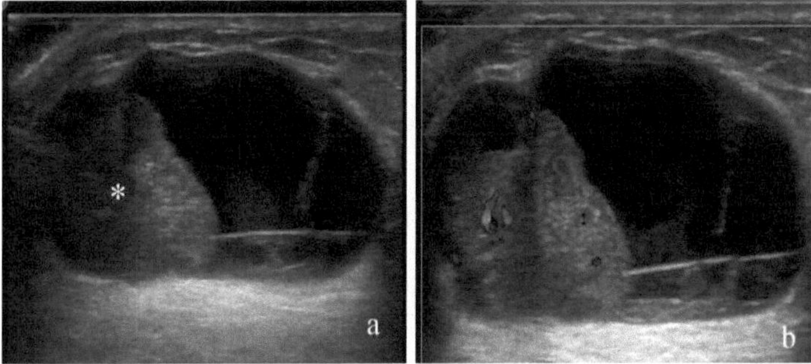

Fig. 52. Intracystic papillary carcinoma. (a) B-mode ultrasound. Solid-cystic mass, with the solid portion showing a mural nodule (asterisk), hypoechoic, with microlobulated contours and the thick-walled cystic portion containing echoes and declivating debris within it. (b) Color Doppler. The vascularized wall nodule in Doppler mode.

6. Invasive micropapillary carcinoma

Breast micropapillary carcinoma is a rare and aggressive histological entity [113]. It was first described as an entity by Fisher in 1980 [114], and it was not until 1993 that the term and classification were introduced by Siriaunkgul et al [115].

6.1 Epidemiology

Micropapillary histological architecture is found in 2-8% of all breast cancers; pure micropapillary carcinoma is uncommon, comprising 0.9-2% of breast carcinomas [116, 117]. The average age of onset is between 50 and 60 years [118-124]. Infiltrating micropapillary carcinoma of the breast is characterized by a unique histological appearance and a poor prognosis due to massive lymph-node invasion, with a high incidence of around 79.6% [125].

6.2 Histology

The histological appearance of micropapillary carcinomas shows massive invasion in epithelial nests surrounded by a clear space within a fibrous stroma. Recognition of this entity is crucial, even if it constitutes a small contingent of a breast carcinoma, as it allows prediction of lymph node metastases and irrespective of tumour size [126].

6.3 Imaging

The mammographic appearance is non-specific, with most lesions appearing as irregular or spiculated masses, hyperdense with microcalcifications in around 66.7% of cases [127-131].

On ultrasound, lesions are predominantly hypoechoic and irregularly contoured [127, 132-139]. In a study evaluating micropapillary carcinomas on ultrasound, 47% of false-negatives and underestimation of lesion extent were observed in 81% of cases [132]. The addition of elastography has been reported as an important tool for better tumour assessment [138] (fig. 53).

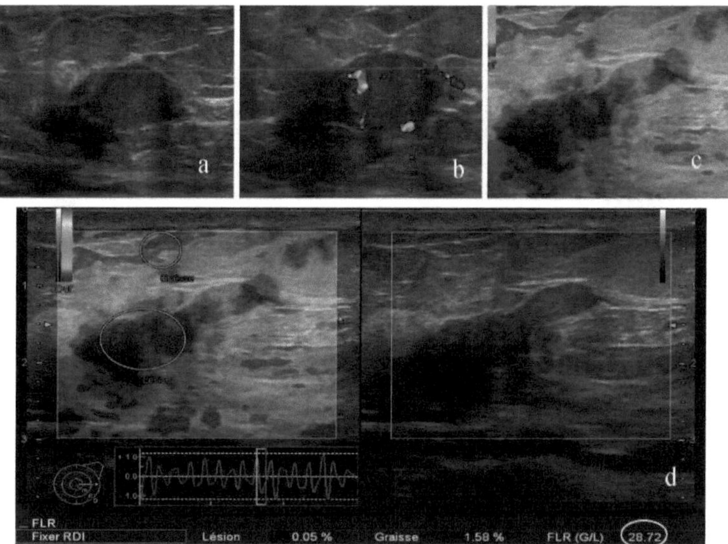

Fig. 53. Infiltrating micro-papillary carcinoma. (a) B-mode ultrasound. Irregularly shaped, irregularly contoured, hypoechoic, homogeneous mass with fine interface, no posterior acoustic effect. (b) Color Doppler. Central and peripheral vascularization. (c+d) Elastography. Hard mass, elasticity score 5, elasticity ratio 28.72.

7. Invasive mucinous carcinoma

Mucinous or colloid carcinoma is a particular histological variant of breast carcinoma. It is a cancer in which the tumour cells secrete mucin. It was first described in 1826 by Geschickter [140].

7.1 Epidemiology

The pure form accounts for 0.8% to 1.5% of all invasive carcinomas [140] and 33% to 95% of all mucinous carcinomas of the breast [140]. The mean age of onset of pure mucinous carcinoma ranges from 49 to 67 years [141].

7.2 Clinic

In over 80% of cases, the reason for consultation is a palpable mass [142-144], often in the superolateral quadrant [144-148].

7.3 Histology

Macroscopically, the mass is soft, round and well circumscribed, with a gelatinous content, translucent or reddish when cut. Microscopically, the cancer consists of trabeculae, cords or tubes, within abundant mucoid patches, separated by thin fibrous septa (fig. 54).

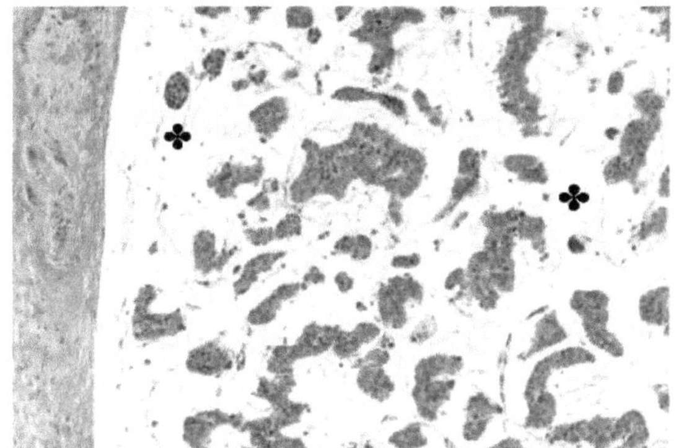

Fig. 54. Mucinous cancer. Microscopy. Clusters of tumor cells floating in sheets of mucus (asterisks) [149].

7.4 Imaging

7.5

The most suggestive mammographic appearance is that of a hyperdense, circumscribed or poly-lobed mass with finely irregular or regular contours [140, 150]. The typical image is known as a "cotton ball", reflecting the tumour's displacement of surrounding tissue without any real invasion [140]. Mixed mucinous carcinoma appears as a mass with irregular or even speculated contours [144, 151, 152]. The number of spicules is inversely proportional to the amount of mucus [144, 152, 153]. Microcalcifications are rare and are usually associated with the presence of an associated carcinoma in situ [140, 145]. Mammography may be normal in 5-15% of cases [145] (fig. 55).

The sonographic appearance differs according to the type of mucinous carcinoma; pure mucinous carcinoma is a lobulated, iso- or hypoechoic, homogeneous lesion with circumscribed contours and posterior enhancement, explained by the presence of mucus (Fig. 55).

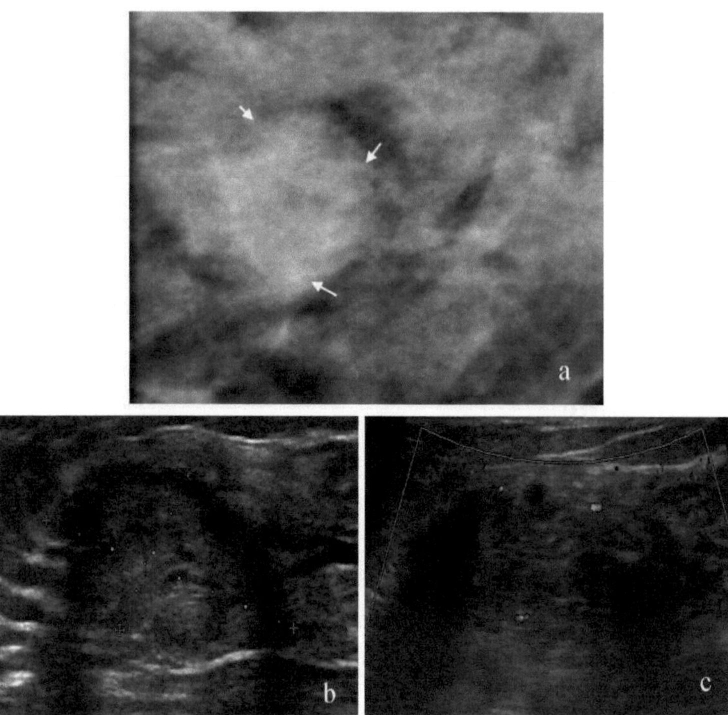

Fig. 55. Invasive mucinous carcinoma (a) Mammogram. Isodense mass embedded in the glandular framework (arrows). (b) B-mode ultrasonography. Oval, hypoechoic mass with microlobulated contours, no posterior acoustic effect. (c) Color Doppler. Weakly vascularized mass.

8. Invasive apocrine carcinoma

Apocrine carcinoma is a rare malignant tumor in its pure form. It is a carcinoma with cytological and immunohistochemical features of apocrine cells in more than 90% of the tumor [154].

8.1. Epidemiology

The frequency of apocrine carcinoma varies according to series, from 0.3% to 4% [155]. Immunohistochemical studies using the anti-GCDFP-15 marker, which is a marker of apocrine differentiation, reveal a higher incidence of the presence of these cells in tumoral lesions, with focal apocrine cells found in at least 30% of infiltrating carcinomas [154]. Numerous studies have found no difference in age of onset between apocrine and non-apocrine ductal carcinoma [156-158]. It ranges from 19 to 86 years, with a mean age at diagnosis of 52 years [157].

8.2. Clinic

Apocrine carcinoma does not differ from other non-apocrine carcinomas. In fact, it most often manifests as a palpable breast nodule, or is discovered during mammographic examination [158, 159]. The majority of masses are located in the supra-lateral quadrant [160]. However, apocrine carcinomas have often been shown to be multicentric in 9.7% of cases compared with other breast carcinomas [161]. For apocrine carcinomas, the rate of occurrence of lymph node metastases is comparable to infiltrating carcinomas of non-specific types [162] and there is no significant difference in ten-year survival of apocrine carcinomas compared to non-apocrine carcinomas, respectively 80.2% versus 78.9% [161]. In the future, the diagnosis of apocrine carcinoma could have prognostic significance with a different response to antiandrogenic treatments [163].

8.3. Histology

Microscopically, apocrine carcinomas are made up of cells with granular cytoplasm, vesicular and nucleolated nuclei, and secretory droplets at the apical PAS + pole. The architecture is tubulo-glandular or trabecular.

8.4. Imaging

With regard to imaging, several studies have found that the mammographic and ultrasonographic characteristics of apocrine carcinomas are similar to those of non-specific infiltrating carcinomas [164-166] (fig. 56).

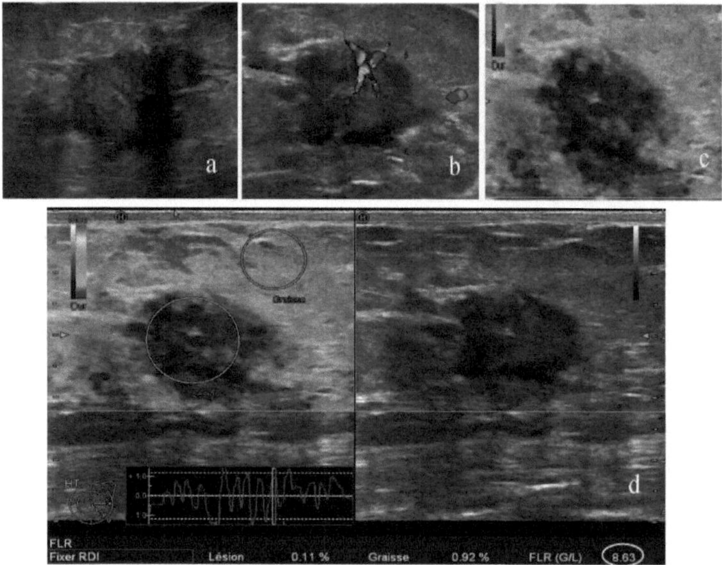

Fig. 56. Infiltrating apocrine carcinoma. (a) B-mode ultrasonography. Mass of irregular shape and contours, hypoechoic, with abrupt interface, without posterior acoustic effect. (b) Color Doppler. Hypervascularized mass (c+d) Elastography. Hard lesion with elasticity score 5, high elasticity ratio 8.63.

9. Invasive neuroendocrine carcinoma

Primary neuroendocrine tumors of the breast were first described by Cubilla et al. in 1977. They are well defined in the 2003 WHO classification by their morphological aspects similar to neuroendocrine tumors of other sites and by the immunoexpression of neuroendocrine markers in more than 50% of the tumor [167].

9.1 Epidemiology

These tumours are rare, accounting for less than 0.1% of all breast cancers and less than 1% of neuroendocrine tumours [168, 169]. Neuroendocrine carcinomas usually occur in elderly women in their seventies [170]. This histological type can also be found in men [171, 172].

9.2 Histology

Four groups are described: solid neuroendocrine carcinomas, atypical carcinoids, small-cell carcinomas and large-cell neuroendocrine carcinomas [167].

Macroscopically, mammary neuroendocrines appear as a round or poly-lobed whitish-yellow mass with a firm consistency, or rarely gelatinous if there is an associated mucinous component [167].

Microscopically, large-cell neuroendocrine carcinomas represent a borderline between atypical carcinoid neuroendocrine carcinoma and small-cell neuroendocrine carcinoma [173]. Cells are large, with moderate to abundant cytoplasm. On immunohistochemistry, neuroendocrine cells synthesize common neuropeptides (serotonin, calcitonin) and other specific neuropeptides such as Neurone Specific Enolase (NSE), chromogranin A and synaptophysin [174].

9.3 Imaging

The mammographic appearance appears to be similar to nonspecific breast carcinoma [175]. These tumours present on mammography as a hyperdense mass with irregular or microobulated contours [176]. Spiculated masses on mammography are rare [177] (fig. 57). On ultrasound, the mass is hypoechoic and homogeneous [176] (fig. 57). Microcalcifications are less frequent than in other breast carcinomas. Skin involvement is rare, mainly in advanced stages [178].

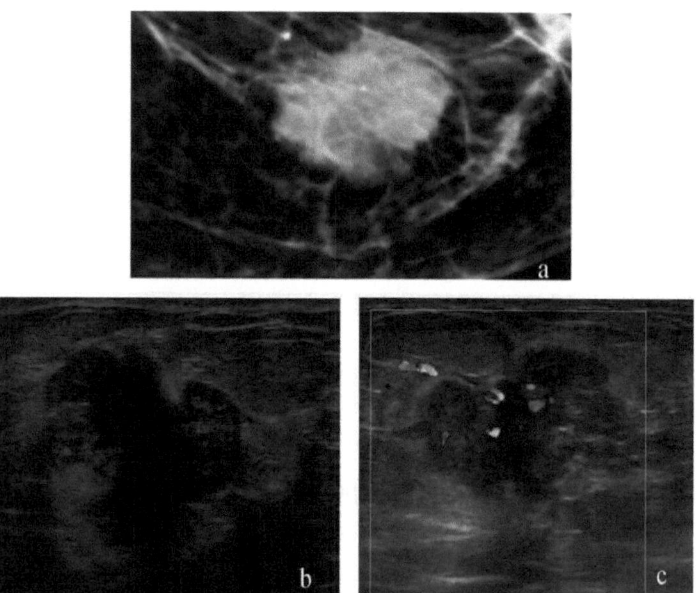

Fig. 57. Invasive neuroendocrine carcinoma (a) Mammogram. Hyperdense mass with irregular shape and contours (arrow). (b) B-mode ultrasound. Irregularly shaped and contoured, hypoechoic mass with no posterior acoustic effect. (c) Color Doppler. Vascularized mass.

10. Other malignant tumors

10.1 Medullary carcinoma

Representing 2% of invasive carcinomas, often linked to a BRAC1 mutation, it is a sharply contoured carcinoma composed of poorly differentiated cells with a moderate to marked lymphoid infiltrate and sparse stroma. On imaging, it appears as a round or oval mass with a circumscribed contour, mimicking a benign lesion [179].

10.2 Tubular carcinoma

Initially rare (1% of infiltrating carcinomas), it is becoming more frequent with the generalization of screening. It is a hard, star-shaped lesion formed by regular cells arranged in tubules, surrounded by abundant fibrous stroma. The imaging result is typically a stellar mass with a very small dense center or architectural distortion, more rarely a round mass or amorphous microcalcifications [180].

Appendix 1: WHO 2012 histological classification of breast carcinomas.

EPITHELIAL TUMOURS	
Microinvasive carcinoma	
Invasive breast carcinoma	
Invasive carcinoma of no special type (NST)	8500/3
Pleomorphic carcinoma	8022/3
Carcinoma with osteoclast-like stromal giant cells	8035/3
Carcinoma with choriocarcinomatous features	
Carcinoma with melanotic features	
Invasive lobular carcinoma	8520/3
Classic lobular carcinoma	
Solid lobular carcinoma	
Alveolar lobular carcinoma	
Pleomorphic lobular carcinoma	
Tubulolobular carcinoma	
Mixed lobular carcinoma	
Tubular carcinoma	8211/3
Cribriform carcinoma	8201/3
Mucinous carcinoma	8480/3
Carcinoma with medullary features	
Medullary carcinoma	8510/3
Atypical medullary carcinoma	8513/3
Invasive carcinoma NST with medullary features	8500/3
Carcinoma with apocrine differentiation	
Carcinoma with signet-ring-cell differentiation	
Invasive micropapillary carcinoma	8507/3*
Metaplastic carcinoma of no special type	8575/3
Low-grade adenosquamous carcinoma	8570/3
Fibromatosis-like metaplastic carcinoma	8572/3
Squamous cell carcinoma	8070/3
Spindle cell carcinoma	8032/3
Metaplastic carcinoma with mesenchymal differentiation	
Chondroid differentiation	8571/3
Osseous differentiation	8571/3
Other types of mesenchymal differentiation	8575/3
Mixed metaplastic carcinoma	8575/3
Myoepithelial carcinoma	8982/3
Rare types	
Carcinoma with neuroendocrine features	
Neuroendocrine tumour, well-differentiated	8246/3
Neuroendocrine carcinoma, poorly differentiated (small cell carcinoma)	8041/3
Carcinoma with neuroendocrine differentiation	8574/3
Secretory carcinoma	8502/3
Invasive papillary carcinoma	8503/3
Acinic cell carcinoma	8550/3
Mucoepidermoid carcinoma	8430/3
Polymorphous carcinoma	8525/3
Oncocytic carcinoma	8290/3
Lipid-rich carcinoma	8314/3
Glycogen-rich clear cell carcinoma	8315/3
Sebaceous carcinoma	8410/3
Salivary gland/skin adnexal type tumours	
Cylindroma	8200/0
Clear cell hidradenoma	8402/0*
Epithelial–myoepithelial tumours	
Pleomorphic adenoma	8940/0
Adenomyoepithelioma	8983/0
Adenomyoepithelioma with carcinoma	8983/3*
Adenoid cystic carcinoma	8200/3
Precursor lesions	
Ductal carcinoma in situ	8500/2
Lobular neoplasia	
Lobular carcinoma in situ	
Classic lobular carcinoma in situ	8520/2
Pleomorphic lobular carcinoma in situ	8519/2*
Atypical lobular hyperplasia	
Intraductal proliferative lesions	
Usual ductal hyperplasia	
Columnar cell lesions including flat epithelial atypia	
Atypical ductal hyperplasia	
Papillary lesions	
Intraductal papilloma	8503/0
Intraductal papilloma with atypical hyperplasia	8503/0
Intraductal papilloma with ductal carcinoma in situ	8503/2*
Intraductal papilloma with lobular carcinoma in situ	8520/2
Intraductal papillary carcinoma	8503/2
Encapsulated papillary carcinoma	8504/2
Encapsulated papillary carcinoma with invasion	8504/3
Solid papillary carcinoma	
In situ	8509/2
Invasive	8509/3
Benign epithelial proliferations	
Sclerosing adenosis	
Apocrine adenosis	
Microglandular adenosis	

Radial scar/complex sclerosing lesion	
Adenomas	
Tubular adenoma	8211/0
Lactating adenoma	8204/0
Apocrine adenoma	8401/0
Ductal adenoma	8503/0

MESENCHYMAL TUMOURS

Nodular fasciitis	8828/0*
Myofibroblastoma	8825/0
Desmoid-type fibromatosis	8821/1
Inflammatory myofibroblastic tumour	8825/1
Benign vascular lesions	
Haemangioma	9120/0
Angiomatosis	
Atypical vascular lesions	
Pseudoangiomatous stromal hyperplasia	
Granular cell tumour	9580/0
Benign peripheral nerve-sheath tumours	
Neurofibroma	9540/0
Schwannoma	9560/0
Lipoma	8850/0
Angiolipoma	8861/0
Liposarcoma	8850/3
Angiosarcoma	9120/3
Rhabdomyosarcoma	8900/3
Osteosarcoma	9180/3
Leiomyoma	8890/0
Leiomyosarcoma	8890/3

FIBROEPITHELIAL TUMOURS

Fibroadenoma	9010/0
Phyllodes tumour	9020/1
Benign	9020/0
Borderline	9020/1
Malignant	9020/3
Periductal stromal tumour, low grade	9020/3
Hamartoma	

TUMOURS OF THE NIPPLE

Nipple adenoma	8506/0
Syringomatous tumour	8407/0
Paget disease of the nipple	8540/3

MALIGNANT LYMPHOMA

Diffuse large B-cell lymphoma	9680/3
Burkitt lymphoma	9687/3
T-cell lymphoma	
Anaplastic large cell lymphoma, ALK-negative	9702/3
Extranodal marginal-zone B-cell lymphoma of MALT type	9699/3
Follicular lymphoma	9690/3

METASTATIC TUMOURS

TUMOURS OF THE MALE BREAST

Gynaecomastia	
Carcinoma	
Invasive carcinoma	8500/3
In situ carcinoma	8500/2

CLINICAL PATTERNS

Inflammatory carcinoma	8530/3
Bilateral breast carcinoma	

[a] The morphology codes are from the International Classification of Diseases for Oncology (ICD-O) [463B]. Behaviour is coded /0 for benign tumours, /1 for unspecified, borderline or uncertain behaviour, /2 for carcinoma in situ and grade III intraepithelial neoplasia, and /3 for malignant tumours; [b] The classification is modified from the previous WHO histological classification of tumours [1413] taking into account changes in our understanding of these lesions. In the case of neuroendocrine neoplasms, the classification has been simplified to be of more practical utility in morphological classification; * These new codes were approved by the IARC/WHO Committee for ICD-O.

References

1. Hill C, Doyon F. Cancer incidence in France in 2000 and changes since 1950. Bull Cancer 2005;92:7-11.
2. Couturaud B, Fitoussi A. Anatomy/surgery of breast cancer. Conservative treatment, oncoplasty. Techniques chirurgicales gynécologie. Elsevier Masson; 2011; 4-7.
3. Lakhani SR, Ellis IO, Schnitt SJ, Tan PH, van de Vijver MJ (Eds.): WHO Classification of Tumours of the Breast. IARC: Lyon 2012.
4. Baur A, Bahrs SD, Speck S, Wietek BM, Kremer B, Vogel U, et al. Breast MRI of pure ductal carcinoma in situ: sensitivity of diagnosis and influence of lesion characteristics. Eur J Radiol 2013;82:1731-7.
5. Hammersleya JA, Partridgeb SC, Blitzera GC, Deitcha S, Rahbarb H. Management of high-risk breast lesions found on mammogram or ultrasound: the value of contrast-enhanced MRI to exclude malignancy. Clinical Imaging 49; 2018; 174180.
6. Andolina VF, Lill√O SL, Willison KM, Mammographic Imaging. A pratical guide. 2 nd ed. Lippincott Williams and Wilkins; 2001.
7. Austin C. R and Short R. V. Hormonal Control of Reproduction. 2nd edition of Reproduction in Mammals, Vol.3. Cambridge : Cambridge University Press. 1984.
8. Faulconer LS, Parham CA, Connor DM, Kuzmiak C, et al. Effect of breast compression on lesion characteristic visibility with diffraction-enhanced imaging. Acad Radiol 2010; 17 (4) : 433-40. Epub 2009 Dec 29.
9. Kinzelin S. Positioning, the √Otape cl√O of mammography examination. Imagerie du sein Elsevier Masson, 2012; 2: 19-27.

10. Mancuso S, Ottolenghi G. The oblique projection in the radiologic Study of the breast. Minerva Ginecol 1989; 41 (7): 325-8.

11. Konguth PJ, Rimer BK, Conaway MR, et al. Impact of patient-controlled compression on the mammography experience. Radiology 1993; 186 (1) : 99-102.

12. Muntz EP, Logan WW, Focal spot size. And scatter supression in magnification mammography. AJR Am J Roentgenol 1979; 133 (3) : 453-9.

13. Corsetti V, Houssami N, Ferrari A, Ghirardi M, Bellarosa S, Angelini O, et al. Breast screening with ultrasound in women with mammography-negative dense breasts: evidence on incremental cancer detection and false positives, and associated cost. Eur J Cancer. 2008 Mar;44(4):539-44.

14. Athanasiou A, Tardivon A, Ollivier L, Thibault F, El Khoury C, Neuenschwander S. How to optimize breast ultrasound. Eur J Radiol. 2009 Jan;69(1):6-13.

15. Weinstein SP, Conant EF, Sehgal C. Technical advances in breast ultrasound imaging. Semin Ultrasound CT MR. 2006 Aug;27(4):273-83.

1 6.Sehgal CM, Weinstein SP, Arger PH, Conant EF. A review of breast ultrasound. J Mammary Gland Biol Neoplasia. 2006 Apr;11(2):113-23.

17. Amersham Health. Encyclopaedia of Medical Imaging. http://eu.aershamhealth/com/medcyclopaedia/

18. Clevert DA, Jung EM, Jungius KP, Ertan K, Kubale R. Value of tissue harmonic imaging (THI) and contrast harmonic imaging (CHI) in detection and characterisation of breast tumours. Eur Radiol 2007 ; 17 : 1-10.

19. Rosen EL, Soo MS. Tissue harmonic imaging sonography of breast lesions: improved margin analysis, conspicuity, and image quality compared to conventional ultrasound. Clin Imaging. 2001 Nov-Dec;25(6):379-84.

20. Athanasiou A, Balleyguier C. New techniques in breast ultrasound. Imagerie de la Femme. 2007;17(4):247-54.

21. Huber S, Wagner M, Medl M, Czembirek H. Real-time spatial compound imaging in breast ultrasound. Ultrasound Med Biol 2002 ; 28 : 155-63.

22. Cha JH, Moon WK, Cho N, Chung SY, Park SH, Park JM, et al. Differentiation of benign from malignant solid breast masses: conventional US versus compound imaging. Radiology 2005;237:841-6.

23. Balu-Maestro C. Basics of breast ultrasound. Imager ie du sein. Paris : Elsevier-Masson ; 2012. p. 101-17.

24. Dickinson RJ, Hill CR. Measurement of soft tissue motion using correlation between A-scans.Ultrasound Med Biol 1982;8(3):263-71.

25. Krouskop TA, Dougherty DR, Vinson FS. A pulsed Doppler ultrasonic system for making noninvasive measurements of the mechanical properties of soft tissue. J Rehabil Res Dev 1987;24(2):1-8.

26. Youk JH, Gweon HM, Son EJ. Shear-wave elastography in breast ultrasonography: the state of the art. Ultrasonography. 2017 Oct;36(4):300-309. doi: 10.14366/usg.17024.

27. Tristant H, Benmussa M, Bokobsa J, Elbaz P. Variation of the normal breast: mammographic and ultrasonographic aspects. Encycl Méd Chir 1994; 810-G-15.

2 8.Sardanelli F, Boetes C, Borisch B, Decker T, Federico M, Gilbert FJ, et al. Magnetic resonance imaging of the breast: recommendations from the

EUSOMA working group. Eur J Cancer. 2010 May;46(8):1296-316.

29. El Khouli RH, Macura KJ, Kamel IR, Bluemke DA, Jacobs MA. The effects of applying breast compression in dynamic contrast material-enhanced MR imaging. Radiology 2014;272:79-90.

30. Wilkinson J, Appleton CM, Margenthaler JA. Utility of breast MRI for evaluation of residual disease following excisional biopsy. J Surg Res 2011;170:233-9.

31. Lee JM, Orel SG, Czerniecki BJ, Solin LJ, Schnall MD. MRI before reexcision surgery in patients with breast cancer. AJR Am J Roentgenol 2004;182:473-80.

3 2.Orel SG, Reynolds C, Schnall MD, Solin LJ, Fraker DL, Sullivan DC. Breast carcinoma:MRimaging before re-excisional biopsy. Radiology 1997;205:429-36.

33. Kuhl C. The current status of breast MR imaging. Part I. Choice of technique, image interpretation, diagnostic accuracy, and transfer to clinical practice. Radiology. 2007 Aug;244(2):356-78.

34. Mann RM,Kuhl CK, Kinkel K, Boetes C. Breast MRI: guidelines from the European Society of Breast Imaging. Eur Radiol 2008;18:1307-18.

3 5.Szumowski J, Coshow W, Li F, Coombs B, Quinn SF. Double-echo three-point- Dixon method for fat suppression MRI. Magn Reson Med 1995;34(1):120-4.

3 6.Sharma U, Danishad KK, Seenu V, Jagannathan NR. Longitudinal study of the assessment by MRI and diffusion-weighted imaging of tumor response in patients with locally advanced breast cancer undergoing neoadjuvant chemotherapy. NMR Biomed 2009;22:104-13.

3 7.Iacconi C, Giannelli M, Marini C, Cilotti A, Moretti M, Viacava P, et al. The role of mean diffusivity (MD) as a predictive index of the response

to chemotherapy in locally advanced breast cancer: a preliminary study. Eur Radiol 2010;20:303-8.

38. Negendank W. Studies of human tumors by MRS: a review. NMR Biomed 1992;5(5):303-24.

39. Bartella L, Morris EA, Dershaw DD, Liberman L, Thakur SB, Moskowitz C, et al. Proton MR spectroscopy with choline peak as malignancy marker improves positive predictive value for breast cancer diagnosis: preliminary study. Radiology 2006;239(3):686-92.

40. Baek HM, Chen JH, Nalcioglu O, Su MY. Proton MR spectroscopy for monitoring early treatment response of breast cancer to neo-adjuvant chemotherapy. Ann Oncol 2008;19(5): 1022-4.

41. Kuhl CK, Mielcareck P, Klaschik S, Leutner C, Wardelmann E, Gieseke J, Schild HH. Dynamic breast MR imaging: are signal intensity time course data useful for differential diagnosis of enhancing lesions? Radiology. 1999 Apr;211(1):101-10.

42. Holland R, Hendriks JH. Microcalcifications associated with ductal carcinoma in situ: mammographic-pathologic correlation. Semin Diagn Pathol. 1994 Aug;11(3):181-92.

43. Rogel A, Hamers F, Quintin C, De Maria F, Bonaldi C, Beltzer N, et al. Breast cancer incidence and screening in France. Latest data available: October 2016 [Internet]. Paris: 2016 [cited 2019 Jul 19].

44. Li CI, Daling JR, Malone KE. Age-specific incidence rates of in situ breast carcinomas by histologic type, 1980 to 2001. Cancer Epidemiol. Biomark. Prev. Publ. Am. Assoc. Cancer Res. Cosponsored Am. Soc. Prev. Oncol. 2005;14:1008- 11.

45. Morgane Sand. Invasive ductal carcinoma of the breast associated with an in situ component: diagnostic evaluation and prognosis in MRI.

Gynecology and Obstetrics. 2019. dumas-02549516.

46. Kinkel K, Gilles R, F√Oger C, GuinebretivXre JM, Tardivon AA, Masselot J, Vanel D. Focal areas of increased opacity in ductal carcinoma in situ of the comedo type: mammographic-pathologic correlation. Radiology. 1994 Aug;192(2):443-6.

47. Faverly DR, Burgers L, Bult P, Holland R. Three-dimensional imaging of mammary ductal carcinoma in situ: clinical implications. Semin Diagn Pathol. 1994 Aug;11(3):193-8.

48. Barreau B, de Mascarel I, Feuga C, MacGrogan G, Dilhuydy MH, Picot V, Dilhuydy JM, de Lara CT, Bussi^®res E, Schreer I. Mammography of ductal carcinoma in situ of the breast: review of 909 cases with radiographic-pathologic correlations. Eur J Radiol. 2005 Apr;54(1):55-61.

49. Wang LC, Sullivan M, Du H, Feldman MI, Mendelson EB. US appearance of ductal carcinoma in situ. Radiographics. 2013 Jan-Feb;33(1):213-28.

50. Chang JM, Moon WK, Cho N et al. Clinical application of shear wave elastography (SWE) in the diagnosis of benign and malignant breast diseases. Breast Cancer Res Treat, 2011, 129:89-97.

51. Evans A, Whelehan P, Thomson K et al. Quantitative shear wave ultrasound elastography: initial experience in solid breast masses. Breast Cancer Res, 2010, 12:R104.

52. Bae JS, Chang JM, Lee SH, Shin SU, Moon WK. Prediction of inva- sive breast cancer using shear-wave elastography in patients with biopsy-confirmed ductal carcinoma in situ. Eur Radiol 2017; 27:7-15.

5 3. Shin JY, Kim SM, Yun LB, Jang M et al. Predictors of Invasive Breast Cancer in Patients With Ductal Carcinoma In Situ in Ultrasound-Guided Core Needle Biopsy. Journal of ultrasound in medicine. 2018,

10.1002/jum.14722.
54. Cong R, Li J, Guo S. A new qualitative pattern classification of shear wave elastography for solid breast mass evaluation. European Journal of Radiology 2017; Volume 87 , 111 - 119
55. Berg WA, Mendelson EB, Cosgrove DO et al. Quantitative Maximum Shear-Wave Stiffness of Breast Masses as a Predictor of Histopathologic Severity. Am J Roentgenol, 2015, 205:448-455
56. Evans, A. et al.Stiffness at shear-wave elastography and patient presentation predicts upgrade at surgery following an ultrasound-guided core biopsy diagnosis of ductal carcinoma in situ. Clinical Radiology , 2016, Volume 71 , Issue 11 , 1156 - 1159.
57. Lanigan, F., D. O'Connor, F. Martin, and W. M. Gallagher. 2007. Molecular links between mammary gland development and breast cancer. Cell Mol Life Sci 64:3159- 84.
58. Greenwood HI, Heller SL, Kim S, Sigmund EE, Shaylor SD, Moy L. Ductal Carcinoma in Situ of the Breasts: Review of MR Imaging Features. RadioGraphics 2013;33:1569-88.
59. Jansen SA, Newstead GM, Abe H, Shimauchi A, Schmidt RA, Karczmar GS. Pure Ductal Carcinoma in Situ: Kinetic and Morphologic MR Characteristics Compared
with Mammographic Appearance and Nuclear Grade. Radiology 2007;245:684-91.
60. Agwalt T, Cunnungham D, Hadjiminas D. Differences in presentation of lobular, ductal, mixed and special typa breast cancer. EJC Supplements. 2005 Sep;3(1):21.
61. Mersein H, Yildirim E, Gulben K, Berberglu U. Is invasive lobular carcinoma different from invasive ductal carcinoma. ESJO. 2003 May;29(4):390-5. [PubMed]

62. David J Hilleren, Ingvar T Andersson, Karin Lindholm M, Folke S Linnel. Invasive lobular carcinoma: mammographic findings in a 10 years experience. Radiology. 1991 Jan;178(1):149-54.

6 3.Silverstein MJ, Bernard SL, James R, et al. Infiltrating lobular carcinoma. Is it different from infiltrating duct carcinoma? 1994 Mar 15;73(6):1673-1677.

64. Watermann DO, Tempfer C, Hefler LA, Parat C, Stickeler E. Ultrasound morphology of invasive lobular breast cancer is different compared with other types of breast cancer. Ultrasound un med and Biol. 2005;31(2):167-174. [PubMed]

65. Colin C. The bloodless combined diagnosis. J Gynécol Obstet Biol Reprod. 1980:104.

66. Guilford P, Hopkins J, Harraway J, Clesd M, et al. E-cadherin germline mutations in familial gastric cancer. Nature. 1998 Mar 26;392(6674):402-5.

67. Maublanc MA, Briffod M. Cytodiagnosis in breast pathology EMC. Gyn écologie. 1989:4-5.

68. Raudrant D, Rochet Y, Frappart L, Cokinos D, Magnin G, Bremond A. L ésions frontières du sein : Etude anatomopathologique, clinique et thérapeutique. Rev fr gynécol. 1995;45:38-43.

69. Lévy L, Michelin J, Teman G, Martin B, Lacan A, Dana A and Meyer D. Diagnosis of mammary microcalcifications. Encycl Méd Chir (Elsevier, Paris), Radiodiagnosis - Urology-Gynecology, 34-825-A-10, 1999, 27 p.

70. Corben AD. Pathology of invasive breast disease. Surg Clin North Am. 2013 Apr;93(2):363-92.

71. Hagay C, Chérel P, de Maulmont C, Ouhioun O, Nodiot P, Plantet MM. Conduite à tenir devant des microcalcifications. J Le Sein 2001; t.11 (1-

2): 79-99.

72. Dixon AM. Breast ultrasound. Indications, techniques and results. Issy-les- Moulineaux : Elsevier Masson; 2009.
73. Arpino G, Bardou VJ, Clark GM, Elledge RM. Infiltrating lobular carcinoma of the breast: tumor characteristics and clinical outcome. Breast Cancer Res. 2004;6(3):R149-56.
74. Li CI, Daling JR. Changes in breast cancer incidence rates in the United States by histologic subtype and race/ethnicity, 1995 to 2004. Cancer Epidemiol Biomarkers Prev. 2007 Dec;16(12):2773-80.
75. Lopez JK, Bassett LW. Invasive lobular carcinoma of the breast: spectrum of mammographic, US, and MR imaging findings. Radiographics. 2009 Jan- Feb;29(1):165-76.
76. Christgen M, Steinemann D, Kühnle E, Langer F, Gluz O, Harbeck N, Kreipe H. Lobular breast cancer: Clinical, molecular and morphological characteristics. Pathol Res Pract. 2016 Jul;212(7):583-97.
77. Jalaguier-Coudray A, Thomassin-Piana J.Solid masses: what underlying anatomopathological l√Osions?. Journal de Radiologie Diagnostique et Interventionnelle, Volume 95, Issue 2, February 2014, Pages 158-174.
78. Chapellier C, Balu-Maestro C, Bleuse A, Ettore F, Bruneton JN. Ultrasonography of invasive lobular carcinoma of the breast: sonographic patterns and diagnostic value: report of 102 cases. Clin Imaging. 2000 Nov-Dec;24(6):333-6.
79. Jones KN, Magut M, Henrichsen TL, Boughey JC, Reynolds C, Glazebrook KN. Pure lobular carcinoma of the breast presenting as a hyperechoic mass: incidence and imaging characteristics. AJR Am J Roentgenol. 2013 Nov;201(5):W765-9.
80. Hilleren DJ, Andersson IT, Lindholm K, Linnell FS. Invasive lobular carcinoma: mammographic findings in a 10-year experience. Radiology.

1991 Jan;178(1):149- 54.

81.Krecke KN, Gisvold JJ. Invasive lobular carcinoma of the breast: mammographic findings and extent of disease at diagnosis in 184 patients. AJR Am J Roentgenol. 1993 Nov;161(5):957-60.

82.Le Gal M, Ollivier L, Asselain B, Meunier M, Laurent M, Vielh P, Neuenschwander S. Mammographic features of 455 invasive lobular carcinomas. Radiology. 1992 Dec;185(3):705-8.

83.Berg WA, Gutierrez L, NessAiver MS, Carter WB, Bhargavan M, Lewis RS, Ioffe OB. Diagnostic accuracy of mammography, clinical examination, US, and MR imaging in preoperative assessment of breast cancer. Radiology. 2004 Dec;233(3):830-49.

84.Wurdinger S, Kamprath S, Eschrich D, Schneider A, Kaiser WA. False-negative findings of malignant breast lesions on preoperative magnetic resonance mammography. Breast. 2001 Apr;10(2):131-9.

85.Kneeshaw PJ, Turnbull LW, Smith A, Drew PJ. Dynamic contrast enhanced magnetic resonance imaging aids the surgical management of invasive lobular breast cancer. Eur J Surg Oncol. 2003 Feb;29(1):32-7.

86.Boetes C, Veltman J, van Die L, Bult P, Wobbes T, Barentsz JO. The role of MRI in invasive lobular carcinoma. Breast Cancer Res Treat. 2004 Jul;86(1):31-7.

87.Albayrak ZK, Onay HK, Karata "g GY, Karata "g O. Invasive lobu-lar carcinoma of the breast: mammographic and sonographicevaluation. Diagn Interv Radiol 2011;17(3):232-8.

88.Cawson JN, Law EM, Kavanagh AM. Invasive lobular carcinoma:sonographic features of cancers detected in a BreastScreenProgram. Australas Radiol 2001;45(1):25-30.

89.Mesurolle B, Mignon F, Ariche-Cohen M, Goumot PA. [Invasiveinfra centimetric breast lobular carcinoma: ultrasonographicfeatures]. J Radiol

2003;84(2 Pt 1):147-51.

90. Butler RS, Venta LA, Wiley EL, Ellis RL, Dempsey PJ, Rubin E.Sonographic evaluation of infiltrating lobular carcinoma. AJRAm J Roentgenol
1999;172(2):325-30.

91. Aoudia *L,* Bendib SE. Breast elastography of invasive lobular carcinoma. Multidiscip Cancer Invest. April 2023, Volume 7, Issue 2.

92. Brklja/çi/á B, Divjak E, Tomasovi/á-Lon/çari/á /a, Te≈° i⁄a V, Ivanac G. Shearwave sonoelastographic features of invasive lobular breast cancers. Croat Med J. 2016 Feb;57(1):42-50. doi: 10.3325/cmj.2016.57.42.

93. Grajo JR, Barr RG. Strain elastography for prediction of breast cancer tumor grades. J Ultrasound Med. 2014 Jan;33(1):129-34. doi: 10.7863/ultra.33.1.129.

94. Boetes C, Veltman J, van Die L, Bult P, Wobbes T, Barentsz JO.The role of MRI in invasive lobular carcinoma. Breast CancerRes Treat 2004;86(1):31-7.

95. Fabre Demard N, Boulet P, Prat X, Charra L, Lesnik A, Taou-rel P. [Breast MRI in invasive lobular carcinoma: diagnosis andstaging]. J Radiol 2005;86(9 Pt 1):1027- 34.

96. Francis A, England DW, Rowlands DC, Wadley M, WalkerC, Bradley SA. The diagnosis of invasive lobular breastcarcinoma. Does MRI have a role? Breast 2001;10(1):38-40.

97. Kneeshaw PJ, Turnbull LW, Smith A, Drew PJ. Dynamic contrastenhanced magnetic resonance imaging aids the surgical mana-gement of invasive lobular breast cancer. Eur J Surg Oncol2003;29(1):32-7.

98. Munot K, Dall B, Achuthan R, Parkin G, Lane S, Horgan K. Role

ofmagnetic resonance imaging in the diagnosis and single-stage surgical resection of invasive lobular carcinoma of the breast.Br J Surg 2002;89(10):1296-301.

9 9.Schelfout K, Van Goethem M, Kersschot E, Colpaert C, Schelf-hout AM, Leyman P, et al. Contrast-enhanced MR imagingof breast lesions and effect on treatment. Eur J Surg Oncol2004;30(5):501-7.

100. Paramagul CP, Helvie MA, Adler DD. Invasive lobular carcinoma:sonographic appearance and role of sonography in improvingdiagnostic sensitivity. Radiology 1995;195(1):231-4.

101. Mann RM, Hoogeveen YL, Blickman JG, Boetes C. MRI comparedto conventional diagnostic work-up in the detection and eva-luation of invasive lobular carcinoma of the breast: a reviewof existing literature. Breast Cancer Res Treat 2008;107(1):1-14.

102.Solorzano CC, Middleton LP, Hunt KK et al. Treatment and outcome of patients with intracystic papillary carcinoma of the breast, American Journal of Surgery, vol. 184, no. 4, pp. 364-368, 2002.

103.Aitbenkaddour Y, El Hasnaoui S, Fichtali K, Fakhir B, Jalal H, Kouchani M, Aboulfalah A, Abbassi H. Intracystic papillary carcinoma of the breast: report of three cases and literature review. Case Rep Obstet Gynecol. 2012; 2012: 979563.

104.Salem A, Mrad K, Driss M, Hamza R, Mnif N. Intracystic papillary carcinoma of the breast. JRadiol. 2009 Apr; 90(4): 515-518.

105. Lefkowitz M, Usar CM, Lefkowitz W, Wargotz ES. Intraductal (intracystic) papillary carcinoma of the breast and its variants: A clinicopathological study of 77 cases. Hum Pathol. 1994;25:802-809.

106. M. Muttarak, A. Samwangprasert, and B. Chaiwun, Intracys- tic papillary carcinoma of the breast. Biomedical Imaging and Intervention

Journal, vol. 1, no. 1, article 52, 2005.

107. Larribe M, Thomassin-Piana J, Jalaguier- Coudray A, Round-shaped breast cancers: imaging-anatomopathology correlations, Journal of Diagnostic and Interventional Radiology, January 2014, Volume 95, Issue 1, Pages 40-50.

108. Gaetan MacGrogan, Diagnostic pitfalls in breast pathology. Case 1. Low nuclear grade ductal carcinoma in situ (DCIS) with papillary, micropapillary and cribriform architecture, Annales de Pathologie, June 2009, Volume 29, Issue 3, Pages 188-193.

109. MacGrogan G, de Mascarel I, Soubeyran C, Barreau H, Dilhuydy C, de Lara Bussières T. Coindre, Approche diagnostique dans les lésions papillaires du sein, Annales de Pathologie Vol 23, N° 6 - décembre 2003 pp. 601 610.

110. Liberman L, Feng T L, Susnik B. Intracystic papillary carcinoma with invasion. Radiology 2001; 219: 781-4.

111. Lam WWM, Tang APY, Tse, G and Chu WCW. Radiology-pathology conference: papillary carcinoma of the breast. Clinical Imaging, vol. 29, no. 6, pp. 396-400, 2005.

112. Brookes MJ and Bourke AG. Radiological appearances of papillary breast lesions. Clinical Radiology, vol. 63, no. 11, pp. 1265-1273, 2008.

113. Bekarsabein S, El Khannoussi B, Harakat A, Albouzidy A, Rimani M, and Labraimi A. Invasive micropapillary carcinoma of the breast: an under-recognized aggressive entity. Oncologie. 12, 54-57, 2010.

114. Fisher ER, Gregorio R, Redmond C, Dekker A, Fisher B. Pathologic findings from the national surgical adjuvant breast project (protocol no. 4). II. The significance of regional node histology other than sinus histiocytosis in invasive mammary cancer. Am J Clin Pathol. 1976;65:21-30.

1 15.Invasive micropapillary carcinoma of the breast - PubMed. Available from: https://pubmed.ncbi.nlm.nih.gov/8302807/. Accessed May 16, 2021.

116. Yang Y-L, Liu -B-B, Zhang X, Fu L. Invasive micropapillary carcinoma of the breast: an update. Arch Pathol Lab Med. 2016;140:799-805.

117. Limaïem F, and Bouraoui S. Invasive micropapillary carcinoma: A rare and aggressive breast tumor. The Pan African Medical Journal, 2021;40(29).

1 18.Stranix JT, Kwa MJ, Shapiro RL, Speyer JL. Invasive micropapillary carcinoma of the male breast: case report and review of the literature. Cancer Treat Commun. 2015;3:44-49.

119. Tanaka Y, Morishima I, Kikuchi K. Invasive micropapillary carcinomas arising 42 years after augmentation mammoplasty: a case report and literature review. World J Surg Oncol. 2008;6:1-5.

120. Vingiani A, Maisonneuve P, Dell'Orto P, et al. The clinical relevance of micropapillary carcinoma of the breast: a case-control study. Histopathology. 2013;63:217-224.

121. Wu Y, Zhang N, Yang Q. The prognosis of invasive micropapillary carcinoma compared with invasive ductal carcinoma in the breast: a meta-analysis. BMC Cancer. 2017;17:1-9.

122. Coyle EA, Taj H, Comba I, Vasquez J, Zayat V. Invasive micropapillary carcinoma: a rare case of male breast cancer. Cureus. 2020;12:10-13.

123. Tsushimi T, Mori H, Harada T, Ikeda Y, Ohnishi H. Invasive micropapillary carcinoma of the breast in a male patient: report of a case. Int J Surg Case Rep. 2013;4:988-991.

124. Dong C-G, Yang Y-P, Zhu Y-L. Invasive micropapillary carcinoma of

male breast with neuroendocrine differentiation: report of a case. Chin J Pathol. 2011;40:704- 706.

125. Gokce H, Durak MG, Akin MM, et al. Invasive micropapillary carcinoma of the breast: a clinicopathologic study of 103 cases of an unusual and highly aggressive variant of breast carcinoma. *Breast J.* 2013;19:374-381.

126. Yang Y-L, Liu -B-B, Zhang X, Fu L. Invasive micropapillary carcinoma of the breast: an update. *Arch Pathol Lab Med.* 2016;140:799-805.

127. Günhan-Bilgen I, Zekioglu O, Üstün EE, Memis A, Erhan Y. Invasive micropapillary carcinoma of the breast: clinical, mammographic, and sonographic findings with histopathologic correlation. Am J Roentgenol. 2002;179:927-931.

128. Adrada B, Arribas E, Gilcrease M, Yang WT. Invasive micropapillary carcinoma of the breast: mammographic, sonographic, and MRI features. Am J Roentgenol. 2009;193:58-63.

129. Yun SU, Choi BB, Shu KS, et al. Imaging findings of invasive micropapillary carcinoma of the breast. J Breast Cancer. 2012;15:57-64.

130. Kubota K, Ogawa Y, Nishioka A, et al. Radiological imaging features of invasive micropapillary carcinoma of the breast and axillary lymph nodes. Oncol Rep. 2008;20:1143-1147.

131. Bandyopadhyay S, Ali-Fehmi R. Breast carcinoma. molecular profiling and updates. Clin Lab Med. 2013;33:891-909.

132. Alsharif S, Daghistani R, Kamberoglu EA, Omeroglu A, Meterissian S, Mesurolle B. Mammographic, sonographic and MR imaging features of invasive micropapillary breast cancer. Eur J Radiol. 2014;83:1375-1380.

133. Romero C, Carreira C, Urbasos M, Martín J, Lombardia J, García E.

Carcinoma intraductal micropapilaren un varón con microcalcificaciones como único hallazgo radiológico [Intraductal micropapillary carcinoma in a male patient exhibiting microcalcification as sole radiological finding]. Radiologia. 2003;45:273-275.

134. Yoon GY, Cha JH, Kim HH, Shin HJ, Chae EY, Choi WJ. Comparison of invasive micropapillary and invasive ductal carcinoma of the breast: a matched cohort study. Acta Radiol. 2019;60:1405-1413.

135. Rhee SJ, Han B-K, Ko EY, Shin JH. Invasive micropapillary carcinoma of the breast: mammographic, sonographic and MR imaging findings. J Korean Soc Magn Reson Med. 2012;16(3):205-216.

136. Michael M, Garzoli E, Reiner CS. Mammography, sonography and MRI for detection and characterization of invasive lobular carcinoma of the breast. Breast Dis. 2008;30:21-30.

137. Kim SH, Cha ES, Park CS, et al. Imaging features of invasive lobular carcinoma: comparison with invasive ductal carcinoma. Jpn J Radiol. 2011;29(7):475-482.

138. Jones KN, Guimaraes LS, Reynolds CA, Ghosh K, Degnim AC, Glazebrook KN. Invasive micropapillary carcinoma of the breast: imaging features with clinical and pathologic correlation. Am J Roentgenol. 2013;200:689-695.

139. Mizushima Y, Yamaguchi R, Yokoyama T, Ogo E, Nakashima O. Recurrence of invasive micropapillary carcinoma of the breast with different ultrasound features according to lesion site: case report. Kurume Med J. 2011;58:81-85.

140. Chtourou I, Krichen MS, Bahri I, Abbes K, et al. Pure colloid carcinoma of the breast: anatomoclinical study of seven cases. Cancer/Radiotherapy. 2009 Jan;13(1):37-41.

141. Komenaka IK, El-Tamer MB, Troxel A, Hamele-Bena D, et al. Pure

mucinous carcinoma of the breast. Am J Surg. 2004 Apr;187(4): 528-32.

142. Benchellal Z, Wagnera A, Harchaoui Y, Huten N, Body G. Male breast cancer: about 19 cases. Annales de Chirurgie. 2002 Oct;127(8):619-623.

143. Giordano SH, Cohen DS, Buzdar AU, Perkins G, Hortobagyi GN. Breast carcinoma in men: a population-based study. Cancer. 2004 Jul 1;101(1):51-7.

144. Kouach J, Elhassani M, Elfazzazzi H, Hafidi R, et al. Multifocal mucinous carcinoma of the breast. Imagerie de la Femme. 2009 February;19(1):59-62.

145. Haddad H, Benchakroun N, Acharki A, Jouhadi H, et al. Colloid carcinoma of the breast. Imagerie de la femme. 2006 Juin;16(2):119-23.

1 46.Ishikawa T, Hamaguchi Y, Ichikawa Y, Shimura M, et al. Locally advanced mucinous carcinoma of the breast with sudden growth acceleration: a case report. Jpn J Clin Oncol. 2002 Feb;32(2):64-7.

147. Cherif IN, El Ganouni N, Dami K, et al. Special appearance of a pure mucinous carcinoma of the breast. Imagerie de la Femme. 2007 Mars;17(1):46-8.

148. Mayi-Tsonga S, Meye JF, Pither S, et al. Mucinous carcinoma of the breast and recurrent fibroadenomas: diagnostic difficulties in a bilateral clinical form. Imagerie de la Femme. 2004 March;14(1):23-6.

149. Boisserie-Lacroix M, Hurtevent-Labrot, G, Ferron S, Lippa N, Bonnefoi H, Mac Grogan G. Imaging-molecular classification correlations of breast cancers. Journal of Diagnostic and Interventional Radiology, Volume 94, Issue 11, November 2013, Pages 1071-1083.

150. Matsuda M, Yoshimoto M, Iwase T, Takahashi K, et al. Mammographic and clinicopathological features of mucinous carcinoma of the breast. Breast Cancer. 2000 Jan;7(1):65-70.

151. Tse GM, Ma TK, Chu WC, Lam WW, et al. Neuroendocrine differentiation in pure type mammary mucinous carcinoma is associated with favorable histologic and immunohistochemical parameters. Mod Pathol. 2004 May;17(5):568-72.

152. Cherif NI, El Ganouni N, Dami K, et al. Special appearance of a pure mucinous carcinoma of the breast. Imagerie de la Femme. 2007 March;17(1):46-8.

1 53.Ishikawa T, Hamaguchi Y, Ichikawa Y, Shimura M, et al. Locally advanced mucinous carcinoma of the breast with sudden growth acceleration: a case report. Jpn J Clin Oncol. 2002 Feb;32(2):64-7.

1 54.Tavassoli FA, Devilee P. World Health Organization classification of tumours. Pathology and genetics of tumours of the breast and female genital tract. Lyon: IARC Press; 2003. pp. 36-37.

1 55.0 'Malley FP, Bane AL. The spectrum of apocrine lesions of the breast. Adv Anat Pathol 2004;11(1):1-9.

156. Rosen' s Breast Pathology. 2nd edition, 2001;pp 483-95

157. Kaya H, Bozkurt SU, Erbarut I, Djamgoz MB. Apocrine carcinomas of the breast in Turkish women: hormone receptors, c-erbB-2 and p53 immuno expression. Pathol Res Pract 2008;204(6):367-71.

158. Benjelloun Y, Chenguiti Ansari A, Benzekri F, et al. Apocrine carcinoma of the breast: case report. Onconews 2006;24:15-8.

1 59.Sternberg S. Diagnostic surgical pathology. 2nd edition, 2004;vol 1, pp 373-4.

160. Rosen PP. Rosen's Breast Pathology. 2nd ed. Philadelphia: Lippincott Williams and Wilkins; 2001 [483-495].

161. Takeuchi H, Tsuji K, Ueo H, Kano T, Maehara Y. Clinicopathological feature and long-term prognosis of apocrine carcinoma of the breast in Japanese women. Breast Cancer Res Treat

2004;88(1):49-54.

162. Japaze H, Emina J, Diaz C, et al. Pure invasive apocrine carcinoma of the breast: a new clinicopathological entity? Breast 2005;1:3-10.

1 63.0 'Malley FP. Non-invasive apocrine lesions of the breast. Curr Diag Pathol 2004;10:211-9.

164. Kopans DB, Nguyen PL, Koerner FC, et al. Mixed form, diffusely scattered calcifications in breast cancer with apocrine features. Radiology 1990;177(3):807- 11.

165. Gilles R, Lesnik A, Guinebretiere JM, et al. Apocrine carcinoma: clinical and mammographic features. Radiology 1994;190(2):495-7.

166. Gokalp G, Topal U, Haholu A, Kizilkaya E. Apocrine carcinoma of the breast: mammography and ultrasound findings. Eur J Radiol Extra 2006;60:55-9.

167. Ellis IO, Schnitt SJ, Sastre-Garau X, et al. Tumours of the breast, neuroendocrine tumours. In: Tavassoli FA, Devilee P, editors. World Health Organization Classification of tumours, Pathology and genetics of tumours of the breast and female genital organs. Lyon: IARC; pp. 32-4. 200.

1 68.Sunita Singh, Garima Aggarwal, et al. Primary neuroendocrine carcinoma of breast. Journal of cytology. 2011;28(2):91-92.

169. Fujimoto Y, Yagyu R, Murase K, et al. A case of solid neuroendocrine carcinoma of the breast in a 40-year-old woman. Breast Cancer. 2007;14(2):250-3.

170. Kim JW, Woo OH, Cho KR, Seo BK, Yong HS, Kim A, et al. Primary large cell neuroendocrine carcinoma of the breast: radiologic and pathologic findings. J Korean Med Sci. 2008 Dec;23(6):1118-20.

1 71.Irshad A, Ackerman SJ, Pope TL, et al. Rare breast lesions: correlation of imaging and histologic features with WHO classification.

Radiographics. 2008 Sep- Oct;28(5):1399-414.

172. Bocker W. WHO classification of breast tumors and tumors of the female genital organs: pathology and genetics. Verh Dtsch Ges Pathol. 2002;86:116-9.

173. Charpentier MC, Qubaja M, Le Tourneau A, Diebold J, Audouin J, Molina T. Diagnostic criteria and prognostic factors for bronchopulmonary large-cell neuroendocrine carcinomas. Rev Fr Lab. 2008;398:63.

1 74.Saint Andre JP, Valo I, Guyetant S. Pathological anatomy of neuroendocrine tumors. Mem Acad Chir (Paris) 2003;2(3):47-52.

175. Wen-Chiuan Tsai, Jyh-Cherng Yu PhD, Chih-Kung Lin, Cheng-Ta Hsieh. Primary alveolar-type large cell neuroendocrine carcinoma of the breast. Breast J. 2005 Nov- Dec;11(6):487.

176. Trabelsi A, Benabdelkrim S, Stita W, Gharbi O, Jaidane L, Hmissa S et al. Primary neuroendocrine carcinoma of the breast. Imagerie de la femme. 2008; 18(3):184-186.

177. Amiraslanov A, Muradov H, Veliyeva H. Brest endocrine cancer. Georgian Med News. 2009 Feb;(167):36-9.

178. Boufettal H, Noun M, Mahdaoui S, Hermas S, Samouh N. An unusual breast tumor: primitive mammary endocrine carcinoma. Imagerie de la Femme. 2011; 21(1): 35-38.

179. Harvey JA. Unusual breast cancers: useful clues to expanding the differential diagnosis. Radiology 2007;242:683-94.

180. Le Treut A, Jeantet B, Boisserie-Lacroix M, Trojani M. Tubular carcinomas of the breast: radio-clinical aspects. Rev Im Med 1991;(3-4):257-60.

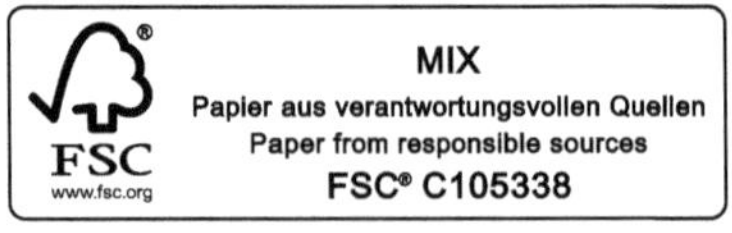

Printed by Books on Demand GmbH, Norderstedt / Germany